Brief Behavioural Activation for Adolescent Depression

of related interest

The Mental Health and Wellbeing Workout for Teens
Skills and Exercises from ACT and CBT for Healthy Thinking
Paula Nagel
ISBN 978 1 78592 394 4
eISBN 978 1 78450 753 4

DBT Therapeutic Activity Ideas for Working with Teens
Skills and Exercises for Working with Clients with Borderline Personality Disorder, Depression, Anxiety, and Other Emotional Sensitivities
Carol Lozier
ISBN 978 1 78592 785 0
eISBN 978 1 78450 718 3

Starving the Depression Gremlin
A Cognitive Behavioural Therapy Workbook on Managing Depression for Young People
Kate Collins-Donnelly
Illustrated by Tina Gothard and Kate Collins-Donnelly
ISBN 978 1 84905 693 9
eISBN 978 1 78450 205 8

Brief Behavioural Activation for Adolescent Depression

A CLINICIAN'S MANUAL AND SESSION-BY-SESSION GUIDE

Laura Pass and **Shirley Reynolds**

Illustrations by Masha Pimàs

Jessica Kingsley Publishers
London and Philadelphia

First published in Great Britain in 2021 by Jessica Kingsley Publishers

An Hachette Company

1

A CIP catalogue record for this title is available from the British Library and the Library of Congress

ISBN 978 1 78775 502 4
eISBN 978 1 787 75503 1

Printed and bound in Great Britain by CPI Group

Jessica Kingsley Publishers' policy is to use papers that are natural, renewable and recyclable products and made from wood grown in sustainable forests. The logging and manufacturing processes are expected to conform to the environmental regulations of the country of origin.

Jessica Kingsley Publishers
73 Collier Street
London N1 9BE, UK

www.jkp.com

Contents

Part 3. The Theory and Research behind Brief BA (the 'Why')

Part 4. Brief BA Session Checklists and Worksheets

Acknowledgements

This manual has been written with the help of numerous people who have supported us over many years. The need to develop Brief Behavioural Activation (Brief BA) emerged from our clinical work with the Child and Adolescent Mental Health team at Berkshire Healthcare NHS Foundation Trust. It was increasingly obvious that the demand for treatment was greater than services could meet. We were aware that this was also a challenge faced nationally and across the world, and that many depressed young people were waiting for months, or even years, for treatment. During that time their lives were essentially 'on hold'. We were also aware that when treatment was finally offered, many young people did not engage well and many failed to complete treatment. Although we both trained in classic cognitive behaviour therapy (CBT) for depression, this was not always working as well as we had hoped.

In our careers we have both been lucky enough to learn from many inspirational clinical psychologists who managed, against the odds, to combine clinical work with research. The scientist practitioner model of clinical psychology that they modelled so effortlessly is one we have both strived to follow. Our role models include Professor Paul Gilbert, Professor David Shapiro, Professor Malcolm Adams, Ms Elin Evans, Professor Cathy Creswell and Dr Lucy Willetts. They patiently and tolerantly helped us to learn and develop our clinical and research skills. They taught us that learning never stops and we are never 'finished'. They helped us face the fears of recording our treatment sessions and playing them back in supervision. They showed us how to use session-by-session Routine Outcome Measures (ROMs) and how to learn from the clients we worked with. Most of all, they helped us to listen and to hear our clients and to never be afraid of not knowing. Many of the basic therapeutic skills we describe in this manual were learned from and with them.

We were inspired to develop Brief BA by the work of Professor Carl Lejuez and colleagues, and were fascinated by their model of Behavioural Activation Treatment for Depression (BATD). This model of treatment was simple, brief and effective, and could be delivered by non-specialist therapists. Carl was enormously helpful, enthusiastically shared his experience with us, and encouraged us to adapt BATD specifically for adolescents.

Working within the NHS team at the University of Reading we were delighted to work alongside a dedicated and skilful clinical team led by Dr Tamsin Marshall and Dr Lucy Willetts. With the support of this team we developed the treatment with young people who were referred to the clinic. At this early stage, Dr Hannah Whitney and Dr Gemma Brisco were essential collaborators, and their expertise helped shape the content and structure of Brief BA.

Since then we have delivered Brief BA in the NHS, in our own university clinic and in schools across Berkshire. This work would not have been possible without the help and enthusiasm of many Brief BA therapists and supervisors who have shared their experiences with us and helped us continually develop to improve Brief BA. We are especially thankful for the input from Jonathan

Totman and Anjali Mehta in their supervision and delivery of the clinical research that has helped us feel confident enough to write this manual. We are also incredibly grateful to everyone in our Brief BA therapist team – Simon Brett, Mona Jones, Michelle Sancho, Alice Moody, Lizzy Hughes, Amelia Durcan, Jeni Fisk and Lizzie Hodgson. Jeni, as a PhD student, was brave enough to try her hand at Brief BA and to take part in videotaped role-plays that have since been published alongside one of our case reports. We also greatly appreciate the input from Child Wellbeing Practitioners (CWPs) and Educational Mental Health Practitioners (EMHPs) across the country, who so willingly shared their views and experiences during Brief BA training. Contributions from all these Brief BA therapists and supervisors have been incorporated into this manual.

Our work was also supported by the wider adolescent depression research team based at the University of Reading Charlie Waller Institute and the AnDY Research Clinic. Faith Orchard has been a constant source of inspiration and support; her creative and innovative research on adolescent depression, the self and sleep problems has helped us shape Brief BA and this training manual. The work of many of our PhD students also features in this manual, and we thank them all – Jeni Fisk, Emily Hards, Rebecca Watson, Sundus Khalid, Monika Parkinson, Iona Lewis-Smith, Simon Brett, Samr Binsaif and Nanthanka Tan. We have also had the pleasure of working with many AnDY placement students; their commitment and motivation to help young people has strengthened our desire to create this training manual for the therapists of the future. We would like to personally thank Tamara Sancho for her continued support on our Brief BA projects as she progressed through her undergraduate studies. Her positivity, enthusiasm and desire to learn have been an inspiration to us all.

We would also like to thank our AnDY Research Clinic colleagues, especially Cathy Creswell, Ray Percy and Polly Waite, who have supported ongoing Brief BA clinical research and treatment in the Clinic and made it such an enjoyable place to work.

This work would not have been possible without the ongoing support of and donations from the Charlie Waller Memorial Trust, as well as generous donations from the Titcomb Foundation Charitable Trust. We are also grateful to the many individuals who made generous donations to the Charlie Waller Institute and helped us pay for therapists and research staff. Thank you all for making a real and positive difference to young people's lives.

We would also like to thank our family and friends who have supported us to make this manual possible, while reminding us to practise Brief BA ourselves and to make time for what matters.

And finally, our biggest thanks go to the young people, parents and carers, school staff and others who have been directly involved in Brief BA and helped us shape this into the intervention you will read about here.

PART 1

INTRODUCTION

CHAPTER 1

Getting Started

How to Use this Manual

Who is this manual for?

- Do you work with young people who experience symptoms of depression?
- Does your role give you the opportunity to offer them a brief, straightforward and time-limited treatment?

If you answered 'yes' to both these questions, then this manual has been written for you.

You might also be interested in this manual if you are involved in training or supervising clinical staff who work with young people who have symptoms of depression and are offering 'low-intensity' treatments.

This manual is designed for anyone wanting to deliver, or supervise delivery of, a brief structured intervention for adolescent depression symptoms. We have pulled together our clinical and research experience, skills and knowledge into one comprehensive guide that will help you navigate both the *how* (the practical delivery) and the *why* (the theory and research behind it) of Brief BA. While this manual is primarily written for professionals involved in offering mental health support to adolescents, some young people themselves, their families or other professionals involved in their care may also find it useful.

What is Brief Behavioural Activation (Brief BA)?

Brief Behavioural Activation (Brief BA) is a low-intensity psychological treatment for adolescents with depression. Low intensity typically means treatment that is relatively brief, that builds on young people's own resources and capacity, and that aims to get young people back to normal functioning as soon as possible.

In Brief BA, the therapist and young person work together to identify how the young person is spending their time (*activity monitoring*), and what personally matters to them (their *values*). With this information they then work as a team to plan and schedule activities into the young person's daily life that fit with what is personally important to them (that is, *valued activities*), to increase their experience of reward from everyday life.

Typically, Brief BA is completed over six to eight weekly or twice-weekly sessions with a review around a month later, and with structured parental involvement[1] at key stages. Session-by-session

1 The terms parent/carer are used throughout the book to refer to any adult with a caregiving role for a young person.

Routine Outcome Measures (ROMs)[2] are embedded within the treatment to ensure that progress is monitored closely and that the young person and therapist share the same understanding of the young person's difficulties and how to overcome them. Brief BA is designed to be delivered by a range of professionals without specialist training, in a range of settings, including clinics, communities and schools.

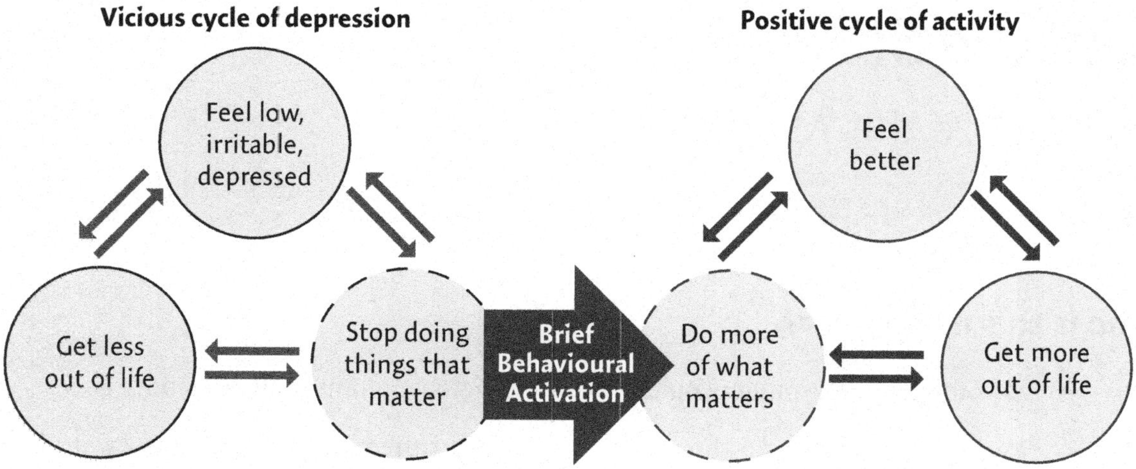

Figure 1.1. The Brief BA model

We often describe Brief BA as *simple, but not easy*. This captures the essence of Brief BA. We have designed it to be as uncomplicated as possible. The core ideas are *simple*. We believe that this helps young people engage with treatment. In Brief BA, depressed young people will be able to understand *why* they feel so down, irritable or empty, and *how* they can start to feel better. Therapists can grasp the key principles quickly and will be able to focus on building a good therapeutic relationship. Parents or carers and other friends will be able to see what might help and what probably won't help. Making therapy simple means that therapists, young people and their parents or carers can focus on working together to help the young person recognize what matters to them, and then to do more of what matters.

But although Brief BA is simple, this doesn't mean that it is *easy*. Depression is hard and unremitting. Tackling the inertia and inactivity that most young people with depression have to live with is hard. Living with someone who has depression is also emotionally challenging and frustrating. Treatment for depression takes commitment from the therapist and the young person. The symptoms of depression actively interfere with treatment. This is why Brief BA is not easy and why, where possible, we encourage young people to use the people who are in their lives to support them. This can be practical, for example helping them get to the next therapy session, or emotional, such as simply listening and encouraging them.

We have developed this manual with the help of young people and their parents or carers, as well as therapists. The treatment can be delivered in different places and we have successfully used it in clinics, schools and community settings. We have trained people from a range of professional backgrounds and with varying experience of mental health. However, because working with young people who are depressed is difficult, demanding and carries risk, it is important that therapists are working within a service that can offer supervision and support and keep the young person safe.

2 Routine Outcome Measures (or ROMS) are used in every Brief BA session to track progress and build collaboration between the young person and their therapist. For more details please go to p.61.

Who is Brief BA for?

Brief BA is designed to help young people who have symptoms of depression. Depression is surprisingly common among young people, but often goes unrecognized. This means that young people who have depression often do not get identified and do not receive any support or treatment. Untreated depression means that they just can't get on with their life, and this interferes with their friendships, social life, school and college work, and family.

Therapists need to be able to recognize depression symptoms in a young person. Importantly, depression doesn't always involve feeling sad or low; depression can feel like emptiness, greyness and boredom. Young people with depression often feel irritable rather than sad. Depression is also linked with increased risk of suicide and self-harm, and this is something all therapists need to be aware of and know how to work with. Therapists will need to be familiar with this information before starting to use Brief BA, so we have included some content around assessment, including assessing risk to self. We hope that it will guide your thinking and help you prioritize what you need to discuss with the young person in your first meeting. Following this discussion, you and the young person will be in a good position to decide if they do or do not have depression symptoms, and if Brief BA is likely to be helpful for them.

This training manual has been written with the needs of a diverse group of young people in the UK in mind. While we hope it will be suitable for use in your particular setting, please be mindful of any cultural adaptations that may be needed. This is something that would be useful to discuss in supervision. We hope it will be useful for therapists who work with young people who have multiple difficulties, including physical illnesses or disabilities, and for those who live in adverse and disadvantaged circumstances. However, therapy can only do so much for any individual. Where there are clear, structural causes for a young person's depression and obvious barriers to their recovery, we urge all therapists to explore ways of dismantling these first. Young people who are being bullied, abused, exploited or neglected need help to escape these adverse conditions first. Therapy may logically and humanely need to wait until the young person is in a safe and secure context, and therefore able to focus on the important task of tackling their depression.

What training and supervision are needed?

Training

We designed Brief BA so that many different people working in a range of professions and contexts could use it. It is not necessary to have extensive knowledge of psychology or expertise in child and adolescent mental health, and no previous training in counselling or psychological therapies is needed. This manual provides a step-by-step guide to delivering Brief BA under supervision.

General training in helping skills

If you have no previous training or experience in counselling or psychotherapy, and especially if your job usually requires you to be 'in charge' of young people, for example as a nurse, or teacher, it would be useful to get some hands-on practical training in simple listening skills. This will help build your confidence, identify habits that may interfere with listening (e.g. giving advice), and give you good foundations on which to build a therapeutic alliance.

Before you begin your first session with a depressed young person, we recommend that you develop:

- Good listening skills – experience of talking, and more importantly, listening to and *hearing* young people in distress
- Warmth
- Compassion
- Curiosity, about this young person, their life and what matters to them
- The ability to collaborate with a young person. In Brief BA, you are not 'in charge'. You and the young person are working together. You need to be able to identify what is important to the young person and how to help them do more of that
- Organizational skills – keep careful records and be well prepared every time you meet the young person and for supervision
- Optimism – depression destroys hope. Offering therapy for depression is essentially saying, 'This can change. Let's change it together.'

Knowledge about depression and how it affects young people

We do not assume that you have any specific training or experience working with young people who are depressed. For this reason, we have included a section on assessing depression in adolescents (see Chapter 2). This will help you recognize depression. It will also help you identify when a young person does not have depression and the 'red flags' that are signs you should seek advice and supervision and may need to refer the young person on to specialist services.

Training in Brief BA

Most Brief BA training is practical. If you want to learn more about the theory and research behind Brief BA, this is covered in Part 3 of this manual. You can also follow up on the references we provide. But this theoretical knowledge is not essential – you can be a sensitive, skilful and effective Brief BA therapist without extensive academic knowledge.

Basic training in Brief BA is in two main parts. First is a specific dedicated training day (or ideally two). This will be workshop-based and allow plenty of time for information sharing, discussion and practical tasks, including role-play practice. Ideally there are two workshop days – one before you start using Brief BA and a second after you start using Brief BA and can bring back real clinical information to discuss, reflect on and learn from. If a group of you in a service, team or community setting are interested in learning to deliver Brief BA, these workshop-style training days can be the most effective way to develop skills, learn from each other and consider how exactly to apply Brief BA to your setting.

The second part of Brief BA training is supervised clinical practice where you deliver Brief BA and develop and sharpen your skills. It is *essential* that during this training period you receive close and focused clinical supervision. You will follow the training manual as described and become familiar with the Brief BA model, engaging the young person and their parents or carers, using the worksheets with them, and using the Routine Outcome Measures (ROMs) to monitor how the young person is doing. Supervision between every session (or minimally once a week) will help build your confidence and skills.

Dedicated Brief BA training days

We recommend at least one full day of training in Brief BA delivered by an experienced Brief BA therapist or supervisor; this must include practical exercises so that you can link the theory to the practical skills. Two dedicated training days allows you to practise more of the key skills and have more opportunity to link theory with practice. At the end of this targeted Brief BA training, you should:

- Know the session-by-session structure of Brief BA
- Understand the behavioural model of depression
- Have practised explaining the Brief BA model to a young person and their parent(s) or carer(s)
- Be able to adapt this to a young person's individual experience of depression symptoms
- Understand the importance of and be able to give the young person positive reinforcement as often as possible
- Be able to use ROMs in a session, interpret them, and discuss them with the young person and your supervisor
- Be able to identify risk and know what to do when a young person is at increased risk of harm
- Understand the limits of confidentiality and how this is managed in your workplace
- Understand the importance of identifying what matters to the young person
- Be able to use problem-solving and contracting to help deal with conflict between the young person and their parent(s) or carer(s).

Supervised training cases

Your initial training in Brief BA is only the start. The real learning begins when you start to deliver the treatment. We recommend that everyone who learns Brief BA starts by working with just one or two young people. During this training phase it's important to get supervision for every session – this will help you plan, review and reflect on what you are learning. Supervision can be given individually, or in groups, where trainees have additional opportunities to learn from each other.

Supervision

FAQs

What do I bring to supervision?

- Yourself
- A recording of the session
- ROMs from the session – make sure you have scored these, and also note any changes from previous sessions. Think about what these changes might mean
- Any problems or questions
- Something to write down any notes
- Reading materials.

Why do I need to record my sessions?

We know that it can feel really intimidating to record yourself doing therapy. We have *all* been there. Most of us hate the sound of our voices on an audio recording or how we look on video – it's cringeworthy and embarrassing. We also hate to hear our mistakes and the stupid things we say. And we may not want to ask a young person if we can record the session.

Despite all these problems, we urge you to record your sessions, every session, to watch and listen to the session, and to bring it to supervision. Lots of trainee therapists 'forget' to record sessions – it's amazing how many times the recording equipment 'just didn't work'.

You need to record sessions because your memory is not perfect. However good you think your memory is, you will remember only part of any event, and we won't know which part you will remember and which part you will forget. You might have a positive bias, which means you will remember the good bits and omit the less good bits. Or you might have a negative bias, and only remember the problems you had, the things you said wrong and the times when the young person and you didn't connect. Either way, you won't learn much. Your supervisor can only rely on your account of what happened, and so what you will learn will be based on your imperfect and biased memory.

During the first few training sessions, get into the habit of putting time aside to watch or listen to your most recent session, reflect on your work and your learning, and prepare for supervision and your next therapy session. Check your understanding of the young person – did you catch their meaning? Did they seem to drift away during the session? Did your speech demonstrate that you were truly listening to the young person?

Supervisors use therapy recordings in many different ways. Most likely they will select brief clips of perhaps one to five minutes. This will allow them to identify and then help you develop your basic listening skills. If you have a concern about something specific that happened in therapy, you could bring that specific part to the supervision session and get direct feedback.

What will supervision be like?

Supervision is likely to be most helpful to you if it is *structured*, similar to the way we would structure a therapy session. An agenda is usually helpful for this. Supervision needs to occur in the context of a good *working alliance* between you and your supervisor (and the other trainees or therapists, if it is group supervision). You need to have shared goals, agree on the tasks of supervision and have a positive bond or relationship. Typically, your supervisor has expertise in a particular style of work or therapy with a range of individuals, and there is likely to be a power difference between you and your supervisor where they are more senior than you. Despite this, you must develop a *collaborative* way of working, just as you will develop collaboration between you and each young person you work with. Developing this in supervision will give you valuable experience to draw on when developing your working relationship with young people.

You and your supervisor will work out a way and a style that is best suited to you, but here are two different structures we found helpful, and that might help you get started.

DIFFERENT TYPES OF SUPERVISION

Case management supervision

The focus of this supervision is to take a helicopter view of the clinical work you are doing. You and your supervisor review your cases as a whole to consider your overall workload. Not every client is discussed in detail, but your discussion may include a quick overview of progress for every case. You will use the session-by-session ROMs for individual clients, noting in particular any cases where progress is slow or where things seem to be getting worse, or no better. Any cases where there is risk to the young person will always be discussed. You will discuss how many sessions have been completed and how many are left, any problems with engagement in therapy, for example if the young person is struggling to attend sessions. Case management supervision will enable you and your supervisor to evaluate your workload and highlight any capacity you have to take on new cases.

Clinical skills supervision

In clinical skills supervision there is time to reflect on and develop your Brief BA skills. This can include any issue that arises in treatment, for example:

- How to introduce and explain why we use ROMs
- Using verbal and non-verbal cues to provide positive reinforcement
- Explaining the Brief BA model to the young person and their parent or carer
- How to increase the young person's engagement in valued activities
- What to do when the young person refuses to include their parent or carer in Brief BA
- Listening skills – reflection, summarizing, checking
- What you can do to motivate the young person further.

The focus of clinical skills supervision will be determined largely by prior discussion and agreement of topics. Supervision will usually involve watching or listening to a brief therapy clip from one attendee, which is then discussed as a group. The style of clinical skills supervision is more reflective than case management supervision. It will involve reflection and observing what goes on in therapy between the young person and the therapist. For example, in considering how to engage a young person in Brief BA the supervisor might highlight how the therapist uses their body language and tone of voice to demonstrate empathy and curiosity.

Ongoing supervision

Everyone who works with young people who are depressed needs to be supported by other professionals. This is true for anyone offering any kind of treatment for depression, no matter how experienced or senior they are. This kind of professional support for therapists is part of 'clinical supervision'. Someone more experienced or senior may provide clinical supervision, but it can also be offered by someone who works at the same level of seniority; this is known as *peer supervision*. The more senior you become, the more likely it is that you will be supervised by a peer, and that you will offer supervision to other people.

We all need supervision of our clinical work for a number of different, but related, reasons.

First, the work is hard, emotionally demanding, yet rewarding. Therapists are first and foremost humans. Therapy is about a relationship between two (or more) people. Being human, and in a relationship with another human, means that all therapists will experience strong feelings in their work.

Sometimes these feelings are highly positive:

- Pride, when you see a young person you work with reach a goal
- Joy, when a young person shares a major achievement with you during a session
- Closeness, when you and the young person you are working with really connect.

At other times, therapists have strong negative feelings, and these include:

- Anger, when the system or the world seems stacked against a young person
- Irritation, when a young person, yet again, turns up late, doesn't do their 'homework', or simply fails to come to the session at all
- Hopelessness and despair, when whatever you try to do just seems to hit a brick wall and the young person in front of you is just not getting any better.

Supervision is an essential way to help therapists handle, understand and manage the strong emotions that are a natural reaction and part of their job. But strong feelings that a therapist experiences can distract or mislead them *and* take the focus of attention away from the experiences of the young person who is depressed. Supervision helps make sure that *your* human and natural reactions do not interfere with your ability to offer therapy, and keeps the young person at the centre of the therapy.

Second, routine supervision for all therapists is essential to monitor and maintain high standards of practice. All young people have the right to receive sensitive, compassionate and high-quality treatment; supervision plays an important part in making sure that this is available. Most psychotherapy or mental health professional organizations insist on regular clinical supervision for all accredited clinicians. Supervision can help maintain high standards in many different ways:

- Therapists who are struggling with their work have the opportunity to explore this in a safe and collaborative space. Supervision can often help identify the source of difficulties and help therapists plan a way to overcome these
- Supervision is a good place to review how each young person is progressing. ROMs are an excellent way to monitor progress and to highlight young people where therapy may need to change or adapt to better meet their needs
- ROMs also provide a way for the overall caseload of a therapist to be monitored and adjusted
- In supervision, supervisors can listen to or watch excerpts of therapy sessions. This means that they have the opportunity to detect potentially non-therapeutic interventions and areas where the therapist could further develop their skills
- Supervision can be used to develop or improve therapists' skills.

I'm supervising Brief BA – what do I need to know?

Supervising Brief BA follows many of the challenges outlined above, but you are likely to be more experienced in delivery of psychological therapies if you are supervising others. Sometimes this can mean you might find it difficult to keep supervision closely aligned with a brief, structured, low-intensity approach. This can be particularly the case for therapists trained in more integrative or longer-term therapies. It is important to remember that Brief BA is a non-cognitive approach; there is no cognitive restructuring involved, unlike other psychological treatments such as CBT.

To maintain fidelity to the Brief BA approach, the treatment should be delivered as closely to the structure outlined in this manual as possible. However, as a supervisor, you are likely to have a greater understanding of alternative treatments and techniques than those you are supervising. We would urge you to supervise Brief BA delivery as intended, while being mindful of indicators that it may not be suitable for individual cases (either when considering starting Brief BA or at some point through therapy). Adaptations should be kept to a minimum and be aligned with the core principals of Brief BA wherever possible. For example, a therapist delivering Brief BA within a school may offer an additional review session after the long summer break rather than try to fit it in around summer exams, while another therapist working with a young person in foster care may offer extra liaison sessions with foster carers and school staff to facilitate information sharing and continuation of support once sessions end.

We encourage supervisors to familiarize themselves with all Brief BA materials, even if they have had experience with a BA approach in the past. It's likely that this adolescent adaptation of a brief form of BA is slightly different from the kinds of BA you might be used to. We expect supervisors may want to know more about the theory and research behind the approach, so Part 3 of this manual might be especially helpful.

If you are supervising a Brief BA therapist or trainee, it's a good idea to have personal experience of delivering Brief BA yourself with at least one young person. If you haven't used this approach therapeutically before, we suggest you make sure that you get this experience first. This means that you can experience directly the structured and time-limited approach, the specific Brief BA techniques, and the personal experience of delivering this.

In Brief BA supervision, we encourage you to use self-practice of Brief BA techniques and to ask every supervisee to regularly bring a clip from a session. Given the focus on embedding ROMs in Brief BA, supervisors should ask about ROMs in every supervision, and ensure therapists understand the expectations around these. If you are not used to using ROMs in your own clinical work, we strongly encourage you to develop this practice yourself. It can be helpful to use some kind of ROM in supervision (e.g. to gain feedback on supervision) as part of this.

Brief BA therapists should be focused on positive reinforcement and modelling; supervisors should therefore be modelling the techniques expected from therapists (and indeed, the young people) themselves.

Want to know more?

As you learn how to deliver Brief BA you will want and need different information and resources at different times. We hope you will be able to dip in and out of this manual to get the information, resources and reassurance that you need. Part 1 (this part) is written for you to read before you start. We hope it will give you enough basic background to know what to expect when delivering Brief BA, and things you need in place to make this work.

Part 2 is the main practical part of the manual. We start by focusing on key information that will be useful when you are assessing a young person, as well as some things to think about before you have your first meeting. Most importantly, we suggest how to start building a therapeutic relationship with a young person and the importance of having an empathic, collaborative and curious approach. We also highlight the key features of depression and how to identify it in a young person. As part of the assessment of depression, we discuss how to assess risks to self (including self-harm and suicidal ideation), and practical strategies to put in place if risk is identified.

Next we aim to answer the question, 'How do I deliver Brief BA to a young person with depression?' We describe the key content of each session and identify the tasks and challenges that are likely to occur. We suggest ways to overcome common difficulties, or at least the ones that our trainees or we have experienced. Your experience will be unique and therefore we won't have anticipated everything you will need, but hopefully this will give you some ideas and ways you might problem-solve your individual challenges. At the end of the manual (in Part 4) and also available at https://library.jkp.com/redeem using the code TAUPAGE we include the session-by-session worksheets for young people and their parents or carers.

As a Brief BA therapist there will be many times when you feel confused and stuck. You might imagine that you only feel like this because you are learning, or inexperienced, or maybe even feel you are not a very good therapist. You might also imagine that one day, when you have had more training, more experience, and are wiser, that you won't feel confused or stuck any more. Unfortunately, this isn't how it works! All therapists, even 'experts', feel confused and stuck some of the time, and this manual won't prevent this from ever happening. We assume that as a trainee or inexperienced therapist you will have weekly (at least) supervision and can find support promptly. If this isn't in place, don't be afraid to ask for it, and make sure you bring your questions and any confusion to the next supervision session.

Part 3 is where we use research evidence and psychological theory to answer the question 'Why should I deliver Brief BA in the way the manual describes?' We take the key aspects of Brief BA and explain how the theory and research support the use of each aspect. Some of this will refresh the content of undergraduate psychology training, so if you have a psychology degree, it will be familiar. However, we do not assume that you have any psychological training – this part is written for those of you who are curious and questioning, as well as for those who have an academic assignment to complete and need to provide an academic background to support clinical work. Although Part 3 is relatively brief, you will be able to follow the references and resources to explore the subject more deeply, if this is of interest.

A note on health and safety

[Please read this before you have any clinical contact.]

- **Therapist:** 'Every community site we work in is different, so you really need to get your head round the set-up for each place you go into to feel confident and safe doing this kind of work.'
- **School staff member:** 'We had an issue to do with school being closed when there was a risk issue, so there are things about the way the schools work that need to be thought about.'

It is essential that Brief BA is delivered under conditions that ensure the safety of both the therapist and the young person, as well as others around them. This is particularly important when working across clinic and community settings where there may be different procedures to follow, depending on where you are. Before you make any contact with the young person, you *must* ensure that the following is in place:

1. A contract or formal agreement to work within the specific setting
2. Confirmation of the site-specific policies that you will need to follow (e.g. safeguarding policies on informing parents of risks identified). This is essential for discussions about confidentiality

3. Completion of any site-specific training (e.g. particular safeguarding training, policies on personal belongings on site, use of child or staff toilet facilities, fire evacuation procedures)
4. Agreed plan and contact details for urgent risk advice from the service (especially how to access this when working remotely)
5. Site-specific named contacts for passing on risk and safeguarding details (usually the named safeguarding leads)
6. Contact details for parents or carers of those young people aged under 18 (in case risk is identified and confidentiality has to be broken in order to keep the young person safe).

All names used throughout this book are pseudonyms.

PART 2

HOW TO DELIVER BRIEF BA

The Treatment Manual

Here, in Part 2, we will focus on the practical tasks involved in carrying out Brief BA with young people and demonstrating the main content of each session. Each chapter deals with one or two key concepts, and we aim to illustrate *how* to organize and deliver each session with the young person. We have used a number of direct quotes throughout this section – these are from young people who have had Brief BA, from their parents and their teachers, and from therapists. We hope that these real voices will help bring Brief BA to life and give you a sense of what the experience of therapy is like.

Some readers will also want to know *why* we do things. For you we have written Part 3, in which we explain the key theory and research evidence that underlies Brief BA, to help you find your way around this and to link the theory to the practice. We hope that this will help you find out more about the theory and relevant research evidence while keeping this section as practical as possible.

There are a few things to keep in mind as you are working your way through Part 2. When the term 'parent' is used, we mean this to refer to anyone who is in a formal or informal parental responsibility role for a young person. This would include adoptive and foster parents and stepparents, and other family members with care responsibilities. Much of what is covered in relation to involving parents can also be applied to other important adults in a young person's life, such as school staff, support workers and close family friends.

We also want to highlight the importance of adapting Brief BA to every individual young person's requirements and context. It is not possible for us to cover every potential variation that different financial, social, cultural and health circumstances can bring to Brief BA, but we hope that this manual will provide you with a solid grounding in the overarching principles. Use your own judgement and clinical supervision to consider how to adapt these to suit the young person you are working with.

CHAPTER 2

How to Assess Adolescent Depression

In an ideal world, young people who experience depression would be offered support and evidence-based treatments without delay. However, young people with depression can be difficult to identify. They themselves often do not realize that there is a way through their difficulties and feel utterly helpless. This means that very often they do not get any support or treatment. During this period, untreated depression makes their lives, quite literally, 'a misery'. On top of their distress, untreated depression interferes with their ability to learn, and with their development and ability to enjoy and experience new and exciting opportunities. Depression, in effect, puts their current life, and their future, 'on hold'.

We want to make sure that young people with depression are offered an effective, evidence-based treatment. This means that therapists who work with young people with depression need to know what depression is (and what depression is not), and be able to identify other common mental health problems.

In this chapter, we will outline some of the key issues you should consider when you meet a young person for the first time with the potential for delivering Brief BA. This is not meant to be an exhaustive list of everything you need to know to complete psychological assessments or to work with young people. We know people will be working in many different settings and it is impossible to cover everything you will need for your individual context. Instead, this chapter is meant as a guide for aspects that are particularly relevant for assessing depression in young people. It should be used in combination with your own specific training, supervision and local policies and procedures.

First steps and introductions

Identifying depression involves much more than simply checking off a list of symptoms and problems. An assessment is your first opportunity to get to know the young person in front of you and to build your relationship with them. It is therefore a critical first step in therapy.

Imagine yourself in the shoes of the young person who is coming to see you. You might want to start by thinking about your own experience of being a young person. It might be a long time ago or just a few years, but most of us can remember some of the key highs and lows we had as teenagers. You might have had periods of low mood or depression or other mental health problems, or had a friend who did. You may have had help with this from a psychotherapist or teacher, or another professional. Or, like most young people who have depression, you might have struggled along on your own. Because up to a quarter of young people will have depression before they are 18 years old, most of us have either had depression ourselves or know someone who has.

Now think about the young person you are going to meet for the first time. You may not know any more than their age and gender. Don't worry, soon you will know much more. For now, consider how they might feel ahead of meeting you for the first time:

- What do they know about you? Will you be nice? Friendly? Will you make them feel stupid?
- What do they expect will happen? Is this going to help? What if they don't know the answer to the questions?
- What's the worst thing that could happen? Will you tell them they're mad?
- What's the best thing that could happen? Will they get better?

Remember, this initial meeting may be the first time they have had any contact with a professional around mental health difficulties, or they may have had negative experiences in the past. It's important that you give them a positive, professional and welcoming first meeting. As a new therapist (or a more experienced therapist with a new client) you probably worry about how you will do. You may wonder:

- Can I really do this?
- What if I say something stupid?
- Supposing I make things worse!

This is completely normal, and a sign that you want to do a good job. If you have first session nerves (and most of us do), use your energy and nervous attention to focus on the young person. Remember, however uncertain and confused you feel, you can pretty much guarantee that your client will be feeling a lot worse.

Top tips for your initial meeting:

- ✓ Explain what will happen in the session so the young person knows what to expect
- ✓ Explain the boundaries of confidentiality – what you will keep to yourself and what you must share with other people (see more about this below)
- ✓ Worry less about what you will say and think more about what you will hear
- ✓ Listen more than you speak
- ✓ You may be tempted to try to write down everything they say – don't do this. Focus on showing your client that you are listening (you will usually be recording the session anyway, so you can watch or listen back if needed).

These things may be useful to consider before you first meet your client:

- Who is invited to this first meeting? Often young people are invited along with parents or carers, but there could be other people to invite who would be useful
- What time or what day should this first meeting be arranged? For the first time you meet the young person and explore depression symptoms, we strongly encourage doing this as early in the day and in the week as possible (avoid a Friday afternoon if you can!)
- Are any adjustments needed to make sure everyone can engage in this first meeting (e.g. physical access needs, interpreter, day or time of appointment)?

- Where will you sit?
- What do you need to bring (e.g. consent forms, audio or video recording equipment)?
- How will you introduce yourself? Will you use any prefix (e.g. 'Miss')?
- What room will you use? How will you ensure you aren't interrupted?
- What will you wear? It's important to be professional, but also approachable
- Is there anything you should be aware of before you meet (e.g. bereavements, conflicts meaning bringing all family members together is not recommended, other potentially sensitive issues)?
- If you are delivering the session remotely, what might need to be done differently and/or thought about beforehand (e.g. agreed method of contact, sending questionnaires in advance, confidentiality/risk processes for remote work)?

How to explain confidentiality and its limits

As a Brief BA therapist you need to hold the confidence of the young people you work with. This is essential for them to feel they can trust you and can speak freely. However, it is extremely likely that occasionally you will need to break confidentiality. The most common reason will be the need to keep the young person safe – if they tell you that they are planning to hurt themselves or have clear thoughts about or have planned suicide, it is important that you are able keep them safe. However, there may be other information that means you have to break confidentiality, including abuse, exploitation or political radicalization.

- **Young person:** 'I liked being able to talk freely.'
- **Parent:** 'My daughter felt able to speak openly about her issues, but I knew they would contact me if they had any serious concerns.'

It is *critical* that you discuss confidentiality and the limits to confidentiality at the *very start* of your first meeting with a young person (and/or parent or carer). This is also something we suggest you repeat at the start of the next few sessions, and you remind the young person of if you need to break confidentiality. As this may feel difficult, you might want to practise in supervision, even before you see your first client for Brief BA. We have included an example to help you think about how you could explain this delicate balance to the young person so that they feel safe and can understand why and when you are not able to keep information confidential. You will need to adapt this to be suitable for you own setting and the individual young person in front of you.

CONFIDENTIALITY (AND LIMITS) SCRIPT EXAMPLE

Therapist: 'Before we start, I'd like to tell you what kind of things we can discuss and keep confidential. What we talk about together is confidential. That means it's private, so I'm not going to tell your parents, other young people or your teachers what you've told me. We share information in our team to make sure we're giving you the best support possible, but we do this in a way that means it is still kept private from other people.

It's often also helpful to share a lot of what we talk about together with important people in your life so they can help support you in the most helpful way, but there might be things you want to keep between us, which, for most of the time, is fine.

But there are some situations when I would need to tell someone else what you've told me, even if you don't want me to. For example, if I was worried about your safety, or the safety of someone else, I would have to share the information to help keep you or the other person safe. Who I share the information with depends on the exact situation, but I might have to share this with your parents, your GP [family doctor] or other adults.

I would always talk to you before doing this so that we could come up with a plan together, like me being with you while you share the information, or me sharing the information for you. How does that all sound? Do you have any questions?'

It is also important to be prepared and to have an idea of what you might say and do when you are in a session with a young person and they tell you something that you cannot keep confidential. Table 2.1 gives some suggestions. However, if your service or employer has specific rules about this, make sure you are familiar with these and that you follow them.

Table 2.1. General steps to follow if you need to break client confidentiality

Step	Action
Remind the young person about confidentiality and limits	Recap what you previously said about confidentiality and its limits Check if any adults are already aware of risk (explain you will need to speak to them anyway – you can't assume they know, even if the young person says so)
Explore the positives of sharing with the young person's consent	Explain that by sharing this information with the adults involved in their care it will help keep them (or another person, if the risk relates to someone else) safe, so you would like to do so Highlight the positives of risk sharing: • Others understanding the young person's difficulties more fully • Not having to keep difficulties to themselves and dealing with them alone • Others helping to keep them safe (e.g. by providing extra support, reducing the chance of impulsive acts by removing access to means)
Explore the young person's view of the potential negatives of risk sharing	Discuss what the young person is concerned about from risk sharing, for example: • Parents or carers 'over-reacting': Explain your training and ability to share information in a normalizing, validating way • Extra stress or burden on the parent or carer: Explain this is part of being a parent and feedback indicates they would much rather know • Any signs indicating that sharing risk information will increase risk itself (this is very dependent on individual context, but can be the case if risk comes from those who may usually be the ones to keep the young person safe)
If the young person consents to risk information sharing	Agree their preferred way of sharing risk, and confirm exactly what information is to be shared, with whom and when Document this discussion and actions in clinical notes
If the young person does not consent to risk information sharing	Explain you have a duty of care to act in their best interests Tell them you will need to speak to a supervisor to discuss what needs to happen next Seek immediate support from a senior colleague or supervisor, if necessary during the session If you are concerned about a young person's ability to keep themselves safe in the *immediate* future, do not leave them alone or let them leave without getting advice from a senior colleague or supervisor Document the discussion with the young person, any input from a senior colleague or supervisor and agreed actions in clinical notes

Some young people will have had previous experiences that make it difficult to trust adults and what they will do with information they share. They may also be wary of exactly who information is shared with, and have strong preferences about this (e.g. preferring information to be shared with their dad or stepmum rather than their mum). Wherever possible, try to clarify these preferences and meet them if you can without impacting on their safety.

- **School staff member:** 'I think the young person was grateful actually that it had been fed back [from the assessor] and it was a bit of a relief that they'd told someone, it was off their shoulders.'

Clinician question: When might I have to break confidentiality?

The key issue is that you must consider the *best interests of the young person*. This means that you need to weigh the risk of breaking their confidence against the risks of keeping their confidence. If keeping their confidence is likely to have more serious consequences than breaking their confidence, you must take the action that will lead to the least harm. You will always be required to follow service and site-specific (e.g. school or college) policies about when this may be needed and how, so make sure you know these policies.

- **Therapist:** 'There was one occasion where I did have to feed back some risk information and the young person I was working with wasn't particularly happy with that, but I explained why it was important and we managed to come to an agreement as to how much information they were willing for me to share. When I talked to my supervisor we agreed this was still enough information sharing to keep them safe, while maintaining some confidentiality for the young person.'

How to assess depression symptoms in young people

Parents, teachers and other professionals are often unsure how depression differs from normal adolescent 'moodiness'. While it is certainly true that periods of unhappiness and some other key symptoms of depression are experienced by many young people, these are usually for brief periods, and the young person is largely able to continue with their day-to-day activities. In this section, we'll cover what to look for with each symptom of depression, and how to distinguish these from more everyday experiences.

A careful and accurate assessment is integral to delivering Brief BA safely and well. If an initial assessment has already been completed and a young person has been referred to you for Brief BA, make sure you have read all the information and associated documents thoroughly, and use this as a basis for checking in on specific issues with the young person and their family. Remember that they may have chosen not to disclose full information previously, and the initial assessment may have been weeks or even months ago, so their current experience might be very different now. Always do a full risk assessment in your first meeting.

Diagnosis of depression in young people

There are two main diagnostic classification systems used worldwide: the *Diagnostic and Statistical Manual of Mental Disorders*, which is currently in its 5th edition (DSM-5; APA 2013) and the *International Classification of Disease*, of which the 10th edition is current (ICD-10; WHO 1992), but the 11th edition is under preparation. Although broadly similar, there are slight differences between DSM and ICD diagnostic criteria and terminology. For example, DSM uses the term 'Major Depressive Disorder' while ICD describes this same group of symptoms as 'Single Episode Depressive Disorder' and 'Recurrent Depressive Disorder'. We have included information below based on the DSM-5 as this is the most widely used classification system, but make sure you are familiar with the way depression is diagnosed and classified where you are based.

Major Depressive Disorder (MDD), to meet the criteria for a diagnosis of MDD (commonly known as depression), a young person must experience at least five symptoms in total, one of which must be a core symptom (low mood, irritability or anhedonia [loss of interest or pleasure]). Other symptoms include suicidal thoughts, sleep disturbance, fatigue, cognitive difficulties, appetite changes, psychomotor agitation or slowness, and negative self-perceptions such as worthlessness or excessive guilt. Symptoms must have lasted for a *minimum of two weeks* and be experienced more days than not, and must *interfere with functioning*. These difficulties should only be attributed to depression when *there isn't another explanation for these symptoms* (e.g. physical health problem, other type of mental health difficulty).

Persistent Depressive Disorder (PDD) is another common type of depressive disorder, previously known as dysthymia. This is a more chronic disorder that can occur separately or at the same time as depression. When someone experiences both PDD and MDD, it is often referred to as 'double depression'. To meet a diagnosis of PDD, at least three of the following symptoms (one of which must be sad or irritable mood) must occur most of the day, more days than not, for at least a year: depressed or irritable mood, appetite disturbance, fatigue, poor concentration or indecision, sleep disturbance, low self-esteem and hopelessness. If a young person has been struggling with depression symptoms for some time, it is helpful to explore the possibility of PDD as a separate, or additional, diagnosis.

Top tips for assessing depression in young people:

- ✓ Explain to the young person that you want to talk to them about what is troubling them most, and although you have some specific things you need to find out about, that you want to hear from them, in their own words
- ✓ Start with an open question or observation. It can be useful to ask something about their own lives to get a picture of this
- ✓ Making an (accurate) observation, for example, 'It seems hard for you to put your feelings into words', validates the young person and shows that you are paying attention to them
- ✓ Explore the core symptoms of depression before checking the other symptoms. Consider starting with anhedonia, by exploring the kinds of things the young person does in their free time (e.g. hobbies, sports, music they like) and move on to whether they have lost interest or enjoyment in these things
- ✓ When exploring low mood and irritability, ask about irritability first before moving on to ask them about low mood – many young people find it easier to talk about their feelings of irritability than they do about feeling sad or unhappy (e.g. 'Do you find yourself getting annoyed with other people?')
- ✓ Pick up on comments that the young person has already made

- ✓ Use the young person's own language when you talk about their experiences
- ✓ Don't interrogate the young person – be empathic, and keep it conversational
- ✓ Use the young person's responses on a depression questionnaire to find out more – it can be easier to 'admit' to a problem when it is written down than it is to say it out loud for the first time
- ✓ Check in with parents – but prioritize information from the young person.

What are the signs a young person might be depressed?

Picking up on the symptoms of depression is not always easy. In our clinical work we follow the general guidance of a structured clinical interview, the K-SADS (Kiddie Schedule for Affective Disorders and Schizophrenia; Kaufman *et al.* 1997). While it is often not possible to follow this in full, the general advice can be used flexibly and may help you identify key symptoms that are troubling the young person. Table 2.2 highlights each of the symptoms of depression and describes how these may present in young people.

Table 2.2. The diagnostic symptoms of Major Depressive Disorder (MDD) in young people, based on the K-SADS (Kaufman *et al.* 1997)

Diagnostic symptom	Things to consider
Depressed mood, *most of the day, nearly every day*	This may be described in different ways, e.g. sadness, crying, feeling blue, down, empty
Irritability, *most of the day, more days than not*	This can be an internal experience as well as expressed as a behaviour. A young person may feel irritable but try hard not to express this (e.g. with friends), and may remove themselves from situations where they feel their irritability may make them behave differently, so others may not notice
Anhedonia: *Most activities are much less interesting or pleasurable. Bored or apathetic most days for at least half the day*	This relates to internal experience, not whether the young person has stopped activities. While young people may stop doing an activity as they no longer enjoy it, they may also still be doing activities but with a sense of boredom or loss of pleasure (i.e. things are less fun). Young people use words like flat, grey or blank to describe anhedonia. Remember interest in hobbies tends to change developmentally, so check they haven't just 'grown out' of it
Suicidal ideation: *Recurrent thoughts of death or suicide, or suicide attempts*	This relates specifically to thoughts about death and should be assessed carefully to separate from wanting to have a different life but still be alive, so explore the meaning behind 'I wish I wasn't here'
Sleep disturbance, *nearly every night*: • *Significant initial insomnia* (1.5 hours+ to get to sleep) • *Middle insomnia* (>30 minutes awake during the night) • *Terminal insomnia* (waking >30 minutes early) • *Hypersomnia* (sleeping 2 hours+ more than usual)	It's important to explore how long the young person is actively trying to sleep, as many will do other activities after the time they go to bed (e.g. using a phone or other electronic device) which should be discounted in the time taken to fall asleep Check in on any practical issues that may be disrupting their sleep (e.g. sounds, light, other people disturbing them), and any substances, medication or medical conditions that may explain their sleep disturbance It is useful to explore how their sleep pattern was before they started having depression difficulties, to assess the relative change (every individual may have very different sleep patterns)
Fatigue: *Tired or lacks energy most of the day, nearly every day*	This is a subjective feeling that lasts most of the day, rather than tiredness from waking early that soon improves

cont.

Diagnostic symptom	Things to consider
Cognitive difficulties: • *Decreased concentration or slowed thinking nearly every day, to the extent that it interferes with school or college work* • *Indecision: Significant difficulty making decisions that impacts functioning*	This should be at a level that is either significantly affecting their academic study or that is requiring them to put in significantly more effort or time This may also affect their ability to follow conversations, TV shows or films, or to make simple everyday decisions like what to wear or where to go for lunch
Appetite or weight change: • *Appetite: Clear increase or decrease in appetite or hunger* • *Weight: Clear increase or loss of weight during mood disturbance*	There may be a change to appetite without weight loss (e.g. the young person is not hungry but eats meals when encouraged by family) This should not be associated with changes related to puberty, growth or recent changes in levels of physical activity or active weight control attempts
Psychomotor changes *nearly every day, observable by others:* • *Agitation: Noticeably increased movement and/or speech, unable to sit still* • *Retardation: Noticeably slowed down movement, reactions and/or speech*	This difference in their body movement and speech should be noticeable to others (including you, as the assessor) and not a temporary change during discussion of something particularly difficult or upsetting. The agitation or slowness should be present for the duration of the time you spend with them (i.e. it is not a sign of initial anxiety that reduces as they relax into the assessment, or tiredness that reduces as the conversation gets going)
Negative self-perceptions: • *Worthlessness: Feels worthless or like a failure* • *Excessive or inappropriate guilt: Guilt over things that are not objectively their fault or are beyond an appropriate level*	Many young people make some negative comparisons between themselves and others, or wish they were different in some way. This reflects a pervasiveness and intensity of these negative self-perceptions, so it can help to ask whether the young person feels they are more critical of themselves than most people their age, or if there is anything they like about themselves. Initial feelings of guilt over parental separation should not be counted here

Note: DSM-5 criteria (symptom information based on the K-SADS; Kaufman *et al.* 1997)

Of the core symptoms, only one, low mood, is immediately recognized as a sign of depression by most people. In fact, many people use the term 'low mood' interchangeably with 'depression' to describe the cluster of symptoms that form a mental health problem. This means that young people who are not obviously sad or unhappy are often not identified as depressed. Rarely is irritability recognized as a symptom of depression in adolescents. This can result in significant under-recognition of depression because irritability is often interpreted as indicating that the young person has conduct or behaviour problems. Instead of people being concerned and worried and giving sympathy and care, irritability often leads to other people being critical, negative and even punitive.

Anhedonia refers to the inability to feel or experience joy or pleasure. This is also less often identified as a symptom of depression. Young people with anhedonia tell us that they no longer enjoy activities that were once fun. They sometimes describe this as being 'bored', as feeling 'flat' or 'grey', and that they no longer look forward to things as they once did.

Because there are so many different symptoms of depression these can be combined in many different ways, and therefore depression can look very different in different young people. Table 2.3 shows how even the same symptoms can be experienced in different ways.

Table 2.3. How different young people can experience depression symptoms

Diagnostic symptom	Young person A	Young person B
Depressed mood or irritability	Feels low, sad and empty nearly all day every day. Cries a lot	Feels irritable when people speak loudly, when they try to be funny, when a teacher asks a question in class
Anhedonia	Some days everything is less enjoyable and some days just some things are less fun. 'Bored all the time' including in class and at home. Gets bored doing anything after 15 minutes	Used to enjoy sewing, making clothes and reading, but no longer looks forward to these activities and does them much less because they've lost interest in them. Also lost interest and enjoyment in most other activities
Suicidal ideation	Thoughts of wanting to kill themselves, including ways to do this, how and when	At night they wish they could go to sleep and not wake up, fleeting thoughts about wanting to be dead every few days
Sleep disturbance	Getting to sleep is really hard, it takes over 2 hours most nights Has to get up at 7am but wakes at 5am, even on weekends	Sleeping more than usual – about 10 hours a night plus falling asleep on the sofa after college, but it never feels like it's enough
Fatigue	It's hard to get going with anything as they have no energy; limbs also feel heavy	Tired all day, even at weekends, even if not doing anything energetic
Cognitive difficulties	Finds it hard to concentrate on schoolwork but also on completing any task, e.g. tidying room, watching TV. Homework takes twice as long and grades are dropping. Is forgetful	Struggles to make decisions. Takes around 30 minutes to decide what to do, which has annoyed friends (e.g. what film to watch, what to have in their sandwich, what to do in break time)
Appetite or weight change	Hungry all the time even though not doing any more exercise and eating more than before they started feeling low	Lost appetite, has to make self eat for energy
Psychomotor changes	Feels fidgety all the time and that they are always moving their hands or legs. Described pacing every day at home. Observed in the assessment that they couldn't stop jiggling their leg and fidgeting with their hands	Feels slowed down, like every movement is slower. Took a long time getting into the room and sitting down. It was observed that their speech was slow and responses to questions delayed, even when discussing light topics
Negative self-perceptions	Feels like a failure and worthless. Hates self and can't think of anything positive about self, sees this as much more negative than friends think about themselves	Most days feels guilty when someone else has done something wrong, even when this is nothing to do with them or when something happens that they have no control over

Actively exploring depression symptoms

Some symptoms can be harder to identify than others. Young people and parents or carers may need additional prompting to identify these specific aspects:

- Irritability: Teenagers with depression may have irritability rather than depressed mood. Many parents and young people will not know that irritability is a symptom of depression and will not think to mention it, so make sure you ask about it
- Anhedonia: Often young people have limited autonomy so may still be engaging in activities despite loss of interest – make sure you ask about their enjoyment as well as their activities

- Self-harm, and suicidal thoughts and actions: These are typically difficult topics to talk about, and the young person may have had negative experiences when sharing this information with others in the past. They may be reluctant to talk openly about self-harm or suicidal thoughts or behaviours. It is important to demonstrate your willingness to talk about this by asking them direct questions. It may take time for the relationship to build before they fully disclose this information
- Hopelessness, feeling discouraged or hopeless about the future, expecting things to always be as bad or get even worse: While not a symptom of depression itself, hopelessness increases the level of risk to self.

Methods to assess depression

Young person: 'It was weird to be asked all those questions, but kind of in a good way. I mean, it was finally like someone knew what was going on for me; they were asking me about all the things I'd been struggling with.'

There are different ways to assess depression in young people, and you are likely to have particular approaches that are commonly used in your setting. Generally, a combination of an interview and questionnaires are used (sometimes at different stages of the assessment process).

The gold-standard interview measure of assessment of depression in young people is the K-SADS (Kaufman *et al.* 1997). This is a semi-structured interview based on DSM-5 criteria and requires training and appropriate supervision to use accurately. Many services use an adapted diagnostic interview schedule, but it is important that if you are using one of these, you check to make sure all the symptoms of depression are covered and you know what questions to ask to get the full picture.

There are also various questionnaires that young people or parents complete that assess depression symptoms. The most widely used detailed depression questionnaire is the Mood and Feelings Questionnaire (MFQ; Costello and Angold 1988), which is recommended in the National Institute for Health and Care Excellence guidelines (NICE 2019). A commonly used brief measure of depression symptoms is the RCADS (Revised Child Anxiety and Depression Scale; Chorpita *et al.* 2000). The full RCADS also assesses symptoms of anxiety so can be useful if a young person has both difficulties. The MFQ and RCADS are free to use and have been designed specifically for use with young people. You can find both questionnaires easily online.

When you use questionnaires to assess depression, it's important to be curious about the individual items as well as looking at the overall score. For example, someone might indicate that they have difficulty sleeping, but when you ask further, you find that this is linked to a medical condition they have and is not related to depression. Some items, such as those about self-harm or suicidal ideation, will need further exploration if anything other than 'never' is indicated. After all, if a young person has hinted that they are thinking of killing themselves, they will surely expect you to respond.

Both interview questions and self-report questionnaire measures may need to be adapted to be suitable for individual young people (e.g. due to language or literacy issues, or other communication needs). There are sometimes validated tools for a specific population you are working with, so make sure you check out the best tool for the job.

What increases the risk of depression?

Depression can affect anyone at any time in their life. However, some people are more vulnerable to developing depression. Factors that increase the risk of depression include life events and adversity, genetics and temperament, and psychological processes. Life events that are frequently identified as triggering depression in adolescents include:

- Problems with other people: bullying, social isolation
- Family difficulties: parental divorce, family conflict, arguments with parents
- Loss: bereavement, breaking up with romantic partners, moving school or home
- Adversity: poverty, homelessness, war, exposure to violence or trauma
- Failure (or fear of failure): examinations, unemployment
- Excessive demands: caring responsibilities, academic expectations.

Young people who have experienced multiple adverse life events are more at risk of depression than those who have had fewer or less severe events. Young people who have a close family member with depression are also more likely to develop depression themselves. Individual psychological processes that increase depression risk include rumination, pessimism and low self-esteem.

The complex network of factors associated with the development of depression means that for any one individual we are not likely to be able to identify the definite cause of depression. In Brief BA we do not focus much attention on the initial cause of depression, but we do give young people an opportunity to consider factors that might have been part of the causal picture for them. In the first session, it can be useful to identify key risk factors they have experienced so that they have a simple causal explanation. Often parents will want to share their views on this too.

Getting parents' perspectives

Parent: 'I appreciated being able to give my own views of my child's difficulties, how this has affected the family and what we've tried to do to help.'

While the young person's own view of their experience should always be prioritized in an assessment, it can be very helpful to get other people's views as well. Parents and carers often have very different perspectives of the young person's difficulties. Some symptoms may be more obvious to other people than to the young person themselves (e.g. irritability or psychomotor changes), whereas others may be harder to see from the outside (e.g. negative self-perceptions). There may be a difference in how a young person behaves in different situations too, partly due to the others they may be interacting with. Wherever possible, try to obtain the views of others involved in the young person's care, bearing in mind that this might not always match what the young person thinks.

It is also important to listen to parents and to recognize their role in helping the young person. They often play a critical part in helping the young person access treatment. They may also be able to provide ongoing support for the young person in Brief BA treatment. One major advantage of including parents or carers in the assessment of a young person's depression is that this starts a relationship between them and yourself as the therapist. It is also possible that during the course of Brief BA treatment that the young person will disclose risk relating to self-harm or suicidal thoughts in response to your careful questioning; this information may need to be shared with the adults who hold parental responsibility. Developing a rapport and getting to know these adults in advance of having such conversations can make it much easier.

Risk assessment

- **Young person:** 'I liked how they make sure you are safe.'
- **Therapist:** 'Asking the right questions really helped identify risk in young people who had never had that opportunity to talk about those things before, so it was not great to hear it, but great to be able to be there to help and support them as much as possible and be able to manage that risk and then think about what the next steps for that person...however, that definitely came with challenges.'

As part of your work with young people, we expect that you have already received some training on identifying and managing risk and safeguarding issues that may arise. However, many people still find it difficult to ask directly about suicidal thoughts and actions. For this reason, we have given some example questions to illustrate how you might ask about these issues (see Table 2.4). We also suggest you keep the following in mind:

- Always ensure you have an opportunity to ask about risk with the young person on their own, rather than with parents or carers present. Often it's much easier for young people to be honest with a professional about these issues, then agree how this information is to be shared with others
- If any risk is disclosed, acknowledge their distress and show appropriate care and concern, for example: 'That sounds really upsetting. Thank you for telling me, I know it's a difficult thing to talk about. We're going to work together to come up with a plan for what might help'
- Use active listening, for example: 'Can I just check that I have understood what you mean when you say…?' (Explain your understanding and check for accuracy)
- Be non-judgemental and do not react with shock, extreme emotion or distaste (you may need to think about how you would deal with hearing this information from a young person so you are prepared). This might also be something to practise in advance, for example in a role-play, or listen to or observe other risk assessments before doing one yourself
- Present yourself as calm, confident and in control (however you may feel inside). Show this in how you react to risk disclosure, for example: 'Let's work through this together to find a way forward'
- Go at their pace and give them time to talk. This may feel as if it is slow and there is lots of silence, but this is normal when sharing difficult information with someone
- Ask the young person what they want to do and plan the next steps together.

It is helpful to let the young person 'warm up' to the assessment before asking risk-related questions, so they can begin to get a sense of the assessment process and feel more comfortable talking to you. To let them know you will be moving on to a sensitive topic, it can be useful to give an opening sentence such as: 'I have a few questions now that may be difficult to talk about but are important for me to know. If you want to take a break at any time, then please just say. You don't need to answer something if you don't want to, but the more information I have, the more I can help.'

Assessing risk to self

Young person: 'It was like "Okay, I can be honest. I don't have to keep this to myself, I can tell her the whole, one hundred per cent." It's just easier for you to speak to someone that you trust.'

Depression is a major risk factor for non-suicidal self-harm and suicidal behaviour, which is why we are focusing on these particular risks here. This is important to remember, but it is not something to be scared of as a therapist, as asking explicitly about suicidal thoughts and acts highlights, but does not increase, risk (DeCou and Schumann 2018; see Part 3 of this manual for further details).

Risk often fluctuates quickly, but bear in mind:

- It is important to differentiate between self-harm aimed at providing some kind of relief, communication or affect change and self-harm aimed at ending life or endangering life. It is critical to explore the aim and intent of any risky actions, regardless of level of lethality, for example, 'What did you hope would happen?'
- The more detached and isolated, hopeless and entrapped the young person appears, the higher the risk is likely to be.

Table 2.4 shows a range of different ways that we have found useful when asking about suicidal thoughts and actions. There is no one right way to do this, and you always need to adapt your questions to suit the characteristics and personality of the young person.

Table 2.4. Possible ways to ask about suicidal thoughts and actions

Type of information	Possible questions
Presence of passive thoughts	Some teenagers, when they are feeling low, have thoughts about wishing they were dead or wishing they could go to sleep and not wake up. Do you ever have any thoughts like this?
Presence of active thoughts	Have you actually had thoughts of ending your own life or of killing yourself?
Intent of thoughts	How strong are these thoughts? (If 0 is that they are there but you don't believe in them at all and 10 being that you definitely want to act on them)
Frequency of thoughts	How often do you have these thoughts? (Once a week, 2–5 times a week, daily, many times a day)
Duration of thoughts	When you have these thoughts, how long do they last? (Fleeting, less than an hour, a few hours, all day)
Controllability of thoughts	Do you feel able to control these thoughts? Can you stop yourself or find ways to distract yourself? What things help?
Content of thoughts	Would you be able to tell me about these thoughts? What exactly goes through your mind?
Intention	Do you feel that you would act on these thoughts? Do you feel safe right now? What stops you from acting on these thoughts?
Plans	Have you ever made any plans to end your life? What did you plan to do? Do you intend to carry out this plan?

cont.

Type of information	Possible questions
Methods	Have you thought about ways to end your life? Do you have ways to carry this out? (Check means for intent, e.g. medicines in cupboard)
Historic attempts: actual, interrupted or aborted	Have you ever tried to end your own life? What happened? What stopped you?
Awareness of others	Does anyone else know you've been having these thoughts? Who? How much do they know about what you've told me? How have they tried to help?

Self-harm

Young person: 'It was difficult to talk about my self-harm but I think it was better to speak about it and get it out there, and talk about what I'm going to do to prevent myself doing it.'

Self-harm is increasingly of concern to teachers and parents or carers, with up to one-third of young people reporting having self-harmed at least once. Repeated self-harm is less common, but still reported by around 5 per cent of 15- to 16-year-olds in the UK (Kokkevi *et al.* 2012). Although it is not a symptom of depression, self-harm is associated with depression symptoms – elevated symptoms of depression increase the risk of self-harm (Heath *et al.* 2016) and in turn self-harm increases the risk for suicidal action (Cox *et al.* 2012). It is therefore important to discuss it in every assessment for depression.

There are a number of ways of approaching the topic. Below the therapist starts by acknowledging how common self-harm is:

Therapist: 'Some young people hurt themselves or feel the urge to hurt themselves in some way, for example they might cut, burn or hit themselves, bang their head against something or pull their hair. Is this something you've done?'

You may want to collect the following information relating to their self-harm:

- What do they do?
- Where do they hurt themselves?
- What do they hurt themselves with?
- Does it bleed or cause physical damage (e.g. cuts, bruises, broken skin, internal damage)? Has it ever needed medical attention?
- How often do they hurt themselves?
- When was the last time they hurt themselves?
- Does anyone else know about it? If so, what did they do, and has it helped?

To understand the young person's experience and to work together on reducing risk of harm to themselves, it is key to identify and address the function of the self-harm: *why* are they doing it, what purpose does it serve? Is there a more helpful (and less harmful) way of getting this need met?

Risk to others

Very rarely, depressed young people can be a risk to others (e.g. encouraging risky behaviour in peers, verbal or physical aggression). This should be considered in the same way as other types of risks, and you should seek supervision about how to manage this.

Risk from others

As part of a comprehensive risk assessment, danger from others should also be explored. Your own service will have specific policies on the type of questions asked and what information is needed to meet the requirements of your team, so make sure you check this before any direct contact.

Other risks

It is also good practice to ask an open question at the end of any risk assessment, to check if there are any other kinds of risk or danger that the young person is experiencing that have not been covered in the previous questions. This also gives the young person another chance to tell you more about anything they may have been reluctant to talk about at the start of the conversation.

Therapist: 'Is there anything else you are worried about, or would like to tell me before we move on?'

When you have completed the risk assessment, make sure you thank the young person for their honesty in answering these difficult questions, and acknowledge that this is not easy to do with someone they have just met.

General principles to remember:

- Risk assessment and management take priority over everything else
- If you have any concerns about how to manage risk arising in a session, seek supervision (it is okay to do this during the session if you are not confident that the young person should be allowed to go home or leave)
- When seeing a young person with their parent or carer, *always* allow time for exploration of risk alone with the young person
- Performing repeated risk assessments on their own only identifies the risk; they do not change it. Therapists should focus on *understanding the dangers* and *taking actions to reduce them.*

Managing self-harm and suicidality

Young person: 'When they said that they needed to call my parents to say about it, it was kind of annoying as I wanted to keep it to myself, but I understood why because it was to do with my safety...and I learned over time that they need to know.'

Managing risks to self can be straightforward and brief, or a complex and evolving process depending on the nature of the risk. We urge you not to be complacent around any type of risk, and to recognize the need to review risk regularly with the young person as well as when you first meet them. The general approach we advocate is that sharing information can help others keep the young person safe, but you need to do so within a trusting relationship with the young person and in ways that help them feel more, not less, understood.

In addition to the safety plan (outlined next), we suggest you follow the risk management strategies outlined in Table 2.5, adapting them to fit the individual young person, and confirming an agreed plan through supervision from your team.

Table 2.5. Risk management strategies and rationale

Possible risk management action	Why this is important
Tell parents or carers that young people are naturally more impulsive and that this is part of normal adolescent development. This means they can do risky things without thinking through the consequences	To help parents or carers understand that there is a biological basis that makes it harder for teenagers to control their behaviour Emphasizes the need for adult supervision and support
Tell parents or carers to remove means of harm so that the young person cannot easily get access to them	Removing access to means of harm is a simple way to reduce young people acting on impulse. For example, Paracetamol is often kept at home, and parents or carers are often unaware that this can be lethal
Focus on what the young person feels would be helpful. This sometimes means parents agreeing to leave them alone when they are upset (e.g. not going into their child's bedroom when they are upset, but texting their child to check if they are okay)	To help the young person feel heard by the therapist and their family To agree a balance of appropriate supervision without intrusive behaviour
Explore the use of code words or numbers to facilitate risk communication between young people and parents, for example, a 0–10 rating scale for mood check in. Agree in advance at what number parents need to intervene (e.g. 'Anything below a 4 needs mum to help me keep myself safe')	There may be conflict or a lack of communication in families that makes sharing risk difficult, and these are hard conversations for anyone to have Giving a short-hand method of communication reduces some of the barriers, and agreeing these with a therapist helps the young person feel their parent or carer will pay attention
Try to encourage the young person to reach out to adults rather than friends, and ensure that these adults have a copy of their safety plan	Other young people may struggle to cope with this emotional burden, and may be experiencing difficulties themselves
Bring any cases where risk has been identified to supervision	To ensure you, as a therapist, have support in managing this, and to explore whether any other input is needed for the young person
Follow up risk management strategies with the young person and their family	To check these have been implemented and are working; to problem-solve any barriers. This information helps evaluate the level of risk

Clinician question: How do I fit in all the Brief BA content if I need to have lots of risk discussions?

It's fine to add an additional session or two on to the total (e.g. ten sessions rather than eight) if you need to take significant time to cover risk management. Also remember that risk management and Brief BA are not mutually exclusive. Brief BA content can include ways to manage and reduce risk (e.g. by engaging in distracting, valued activities as an alternative to self-harm, connecting with others who can help support them to stay safe). It is important that all the Brief BA content is covered, but this should not be done while compromising risk management – make this clear to the family so they understand how many extra sessions are scheduled if this is needed, and what is expected (e.g. if an additional session is needed early on, Session 6 might not cover Session 6 content, and so might not involve parents).

How to collaboratively create a safety plan

■ **Young person:** 'It's reduced my urges of self-harm, because it's given me ways to cope with it...and I feel able to stop before it gets to the point where it's a lot of damage.'

The session worksheets contain a safety plan to be completed with the young person. This is a short, practical plan that is filled out collaboratively between the therapist and young person, using the young person's own ideas on how to get support and keep safe. The safety plan should include what they can do for themselves, and from whom and where they can get support. Wherever possible, the content of the safety plan should come from the young person themselves, so the plans that are included are ones they are comfortable with. Sometimes you may need to give them information about additional strategies they were not aware of or hadn't considered before (e.g. self-soothing activities, crisis services, anonymous helplines).

Safety plans can be used at any time a young person feels overwhelmed, angry, irritable or distressed, even if they do not have suicidal ideation or feel an urge to self-harm. Safety plans should be tailored to the individual risks and related safety behaviours for the young person you are working with (e.g. if they have an urge to cut with a razor blade, they may agree to parents keeping hold of razors), and the context they are in (e.g. support from parents may not be possible if this is not a safe relationship). It is easiest to create a safety plan when a young person is not in significant distress; however, you may need to help the young person to create a safety plan when they are in distress and at risk.

Red flags: Issues that should be taken to supervision

■ **Therapist:** 'Supervision was absolutely vital in my Brief BA work – it helped me to talk through any risk issues that came up, feel supported, and agree a plan that felt appropriate.'

Any concerns about a young person, regardless of what stage of assessment or therapy you are at, should always be taken to supervision. You should never feel as if you are holding a burden of responsibility alone; good therapists make use of supervision to share their concerns and consider best courses of action. Seeking supervision can be done at any time and for any reason within your Brief BA work, but there are some issues that are particular indicators of the need to discuss with your supervisor (see Table 2.6).

Table 2.6. Issues to take to supervision

Issue	Why this should be taken to supervision
Every new case	To consider any particular challenges or opportunities for this case at the start of the work; to ensure your supervisor is aware they are on your caseload
Any risk identified	To support you in managing this, to consider the risk management plan and if additional input is required
Young person or parent or carer is evasive when discussing risk information	May indicate a greater level of risk than is being disclosed; limited engagement in risk discussions may constitute increased risk (e.g. safety plan not being implemented)
Any indication that the young person is not willing to share risk information with parents or carers	Need to consider the balance between sharing information versus the therapeutic relationship when considering breaking confidentiality without the young person's consent Note: This should be discussed immediately if there is known risk and the young person does not consent to share. Seek immediate guidance from your supervisor

cont.

Issue	Why this should be taken to supervision
Drugs, alcohol or substance misuse	May need specialist input
Behaviour that is disorganized, suspicious, chaotic, out of the ordinary, socially withdrawn, or otherwise strange	May indicate substance misuse, psychotic symptoms and/or neurological issues
Non-attendance at sessions	Need for more assertive outreach May indicate difficulties in the therapeutic alliance that need addressing
Hostility or conflict between young person and parents or carers in session	This is likely to undermine treatment; may need to have separate sessions with adults May also indicate safeguarding issues
Any digital or online activity that you are not confident is safe or supervised appropriately	May indicate grooming or radicalization or exposure to material that is not age-appropriate
Young person mentions relationships with older individuals without clear indication that their family is aware and are carefully monitoring this	May indicate power imbalance, exposure to experiences that are not age-appropriate, and potentially sexual activity that may not be legal and could indicate an abuse of power
Physical health condition or medication issues	May need to signpost the young person to additional input (e.g. family doctor), or adapt therapy to take this into account (e.g. medication leading to drowsiness in morning, unable to engage in some valued activities)
Any diversity issues that are identified	Issues relating to culture, spirituality, race or ethnicity, disability, gender, sexuality, or other diversity should be considered in therapy. Supervision provides a space to consider if therapy needs to be adapted (e.g. in some religions and cultures suicidal ideation is completely taboo; clash between the young person's sexuality and their parents' or carers' views on this may be an underlying conflict between them)

Looking after yourself

- **Therapist:** 'It can be exhausting for all parties...it's what we have to do, I know it's our job, but it's just kind of a lot and it can be pretty stressful; it can be distressing depending on what the risk is, depending on how the young person and parents respond, and just managing that is pretty difficult.'

Asking young people about depression symptoms, self-harm and suicidal thoughts and actions can be hugely beneficial for the individual. This may be the first time they have had a supportive adult wanting to understand their experience and to help them manage these difficulties. However, it's important to recognize that this can be difficult for any professional, especially if they have less experience or training (although this challenge never goes away completely). You will need to look after yourself to make sure you are in the best position you can be to help.

Looking after yourself is an important skill to develop as a therapist, as in order to support someone else, you need to support yourself too. Self-care is key when engaging in any clinical work, a bit like putting on your own oxygen mask first so you can help someone else. It can be even more important when working with depression, where you can feel the personal relevance of experiences of loss or failure that your client is telling you about. There are also often lots of negative feelings expressed in depression assessment and therapy sessions that can affect your own feelings (an effect called 'emotional contagion'). This is understandable – if you are working with someone who is feeling hopeless and that things will never change, it can be easy to start to feel that way too. It can be particularly difficult to hear hopelessness expressed by a young person. Adolescence is meant to be the 'happiest time of your life', or so people are led to believe. It can also be very distressing to hear about negative experiences that some young people will have had, and to witness how distressed and debilitated they are by their depression symptoms. This all means that you need to have good self-care strategies in place before you start your clinical work, and make sure these are embedded into your regular schedule and activities.

Things you can do to look after yourself:

- Have regular supervision, and seek immediate supervision for any risk issue that you want a second opinion on
- Recognize what is beyond your ability and/or professional capacity to manage
- Acknowledge that working with depressed young people can be hard and upsetting at times, and it's okay to feel that way
- Be honest about your limits. Every professional working with young people has their own sense of what they are able to manage, and so it's important you don't try to push yourself past this
- Give yourself enough time between appointments where you anticipate there might be risk discussions and actions needed, to make sure you aren't rushed
- Consider your caseload and whether you have enough resources to manage risk for every young person you are working with, in the time that you have available
- Discuss with your supervisor and team about any additional training that might be useful to improve skills and confidence in managing self-harm and suicidality in young people
- If you are feeling overwhelmed, share this with others
- Use Brief BA yourself as self-practice (see below).

Brief BA self-practice

Therapist: 'I found doing Brief BA myself was incredibly helpful for learning the techniques, but most importantly it gave me a new appreciation of how it might feel for the young people I work with.'

We strongly encourage anyone who is thinking about delivering or supervising Brief BA to try out the techniques themselves as self-practice before starting with a young person. This is for many reasons, including:

- In order to teach a skill, you need to master it yourself first
- Doing your own 'homework' gives you a much greater appreciation of the challenges and barriers involved, and how to overcome them

- Having personal experience with the Brief BA material will help you explain the approach in a more genuine way
- Personally experiencing the effect that making small behavioural changes that link with your own personal values has on your own mood will help you gain confidence that this simple, straightforward approach can be very powerful
- Exploring your own values will give you greater self-awareness of how these affect your assumptions and views of other people's values, including those of young people
- Brief BA aims to increase an individual's experience of reward from life, so it should enhance your own wellbeing and help buffer against the emotional impact of working with depressed young people.

Often the most successful way to try out Brief BA on yourself is to do so with a formal or informal peer group, so you can plan activities and discuss the process together. This can work well by setting up a peer supervision group in your team, where you meet to agree how to try out a specific Brief BA aspect, set your own homework tasks, then meet at an agreed future date to review how this went. It's not necessary to discuss the personal content of all the Brief BA strategies (you don't need to share your personal values or valued activities with everyone), but having a sense of accountability to report back to others helps mirror the experience of having a therapist checking in with you on tasks you agreed to. It also means you can learn more quickly, hearing other people's experiences that may be relevant to the young people you will be working with.

If you do not have time or the resources to complete the full Brief BA package yourself, we suggest that as a minimum you try these techniques:

- Complete your own activity log and set this as 'homework' for yourself (it's surprising how easy it is to forget!). It is particularly helpful to cover both work and non-work days as well as different types of work days if your daily routine changes between them
- Review your own activity log for Achievement, Closeness, Enjoyment and Importance
- Complete your own values worksheet
- Plan, schedule, complete and review valued activities linked to one or more values you would like to do more towards
- Review how engaging in valued activities affects your mood and overall wellbeing.

Some people can find this process of self-practice rather confronting, especially if there is an area of their life in which they are unhappy or facing significant challenges. We still encourage you to try Brief BA out if you are feeling like this, as it will give you a framework to consider how you can increase the experience of reward from your everyday life, even in small ways.

Top tips: Questions that may be useful to consider within your own self-practice of Brief BA:

- ✓ What got in the way of me completing my 'homework'? How can I increase the chance of remembering? How might this be similar or different for depressed young people?
- ✓ How does what I do affect how I feel on a day-to-day basis? What's missing in my activity log and where can I add more reward into my life? Are there 'quick wins' or obvious opportunities? How might I be able to help a young person explore their activity log to identify these?

✓ How did it feel thinking about my values, and putting them on paper? What would help me feel honest enough to share these with someone else? How can I help a young person feel okay about sharing this?

✓ How can I break valued activities into smaller steps to make them achievable? How small is small enough? How might I need to reduce this even further when planning activities with a depressed young person?

✓ What helps me engage in a valued activity, and how can I use this experience to make me a better Brief BA therapist? How can I bring valued activities into my sessions?

Suitability for Brief BA

It is likely that most young people with depression symptoms may find Brief BA helpful, either as a standalone treatment or in combination with other interventions (e.g. anti-depressant medication). Brief BA can also be an excellent starting point for longer-term psychological treatment with a young person. However, there are some young people for whom a brief intervention is not the most helpful. A young person who has long-term difficulties with emotion regulation, a significant trauma history or other experiences that make it hard for them to engage in a short, structured piece of psychological work with a new person is likely to need longer-term therapy to build a trusting relationship in which to develop some of these skills.

Suitability for Brief BA should always be considered in the context of your specific setting (there are likely to be certain inclusion and exclusion criteria you will need to adhere to), but these questions can help you with the decision-making around Brief BA:

- Is this young person in crisis? If so, they need specialist, immediate support (e.g. a crisis team, urgent psychiatrist appointment, going to hospital to keep themselves safe)
- Is there a need for medication? If so, this may not be something that's available in your team
- Is something else more urgent that should be dealt with before the depression symptoms? For example, an eating disorder, active psychosis symptoms that put the young person in danger
- Does this young person need non-mental health support first? For some young people, the most helpful intervention might not be around mental health but focused on improving their living conditions, removing them from an abusive environment or obtaining financial assistance to tackle poverty that is affecting all aspects of their lives. Anyone would find these conditions difficult, so it's important not to frame these as mental health difficulties
- Is there another mental health difficulty the young person wants help with first? Anxiety is the most common of these.

Most young people who are depressed also have difficulties with anxiety. It's not always easy to decide which one to focus on as a starting point, but young people themselves will often have an idea about which is the biggest problem, or where they want to start. For some young people, their depression symptoms have emerged as a result of avoiding things because of anxiety; they therefore believe that if they were less anxious, their mood would also improve. Other young people may feel that facing their fears in anxiety treatment is too difficult with their current depression symptoms, and they need to work on depression first. Treatment decisions should always be discussed with the young person collaboratively and taken to supervision.

Clinician question: What if I'm working with a very complex case? Isn't this approach too simple?

> Not necessarily. The evidence suggests that for adults with severe symptoms of depression, Brief BA might be more effective than longer and more complex psychological therapies, such as CBT. This might be because the simple and practical message of BA and the therapy itself is easier to understand than more complicated treatments.

The Brief BA focused and structured approach can also be used alongside additional interventions as necessary. If other professionals are involved, for example a child psychiatrist is working with the young person to monitor medication, make sure that they have a clear understanding of the Brief BA approach. Using ROMs and eliciting feedback from the young person at every session means that you can regularly review progress, and this can help prompt discussions about alternative treatment approaches with your supervisor and the wider clinical team if progress is slow or if no progress is being made.

Introducing Brief BA as a treatment option

- **Therapist:** 'Brief BA is a practical, straightforward treatment based on helping you understand what matters to you, then doing more of what matters in your day-to-day life.'
- **Parent:** 'I like the principle of Brief BA. Most of it seems common sense and the sort of thing you would try anyway. As a parent, this is exactly the type of thing you would try and do with someone struggling like this. But having that other adult go through this with your teenager makes a huge difference. They will listen to another adult when they won't listen to a parent.'

Once you have completed your assessment and discussed this information with your supervisor, you will have an idea of whether it feels suitable to offer Brief BA as a treatment option. For young people where it seems suitable, you will want to introduce the idea of Brief BA to give them and their families enough information to decide whether they think this type of therapy will be right for them. This helps a young person understand what to expect in Brief BA treatment, and what is expected of them. Parents, carers and other adults involved in the young person's life also find it useful to understand more about the treatment approach before they are asked to help support the work.

As Brief BA is based on a straightforward idea ('Do more of what matters to you'), the rationale can be easily shared and explained so others understand what is involved. As discussion of treatment options can often happen at the end of what can be a long and draining assessment process, it's helpful to share some written material so young people, parents or carers can take this away to read later. You can download information about Brief BA that has been written for young people and their parents at https://library.jkp.com/redeem using the code TAUPAGE, and there are copies of information leaflets for young people and parents in Part 4 of this manual.

It is important that young people understand what Brief BA involves, and that they are willing to give it a try (even if they are not sure it will help) before they feel like they are signed up for the treatment. This is the first step towards a collaborative, therapeutic relationship between you and them.

Structure and timing of Brief BA sessions

Brief BA is a structured, manualized intervention. While there is flexibility in how and when sessions are delivered, most people will find it helpful to stick to the outline shown below, as this is how the worksheets are laid out, and we have found this order of content works well for most young people. Each Brief BA session is designed to be up to an hour long (assuming an assessment has already been completed, including a comprehensive risk assessment and a safety management plan, as required).

OVERVIEW OF BRIEF BA SESSIONS

1. Session 1 (+P): **Brief BA rationale, activity log**
2. Session 2: Review activity log, balance of activities
3. Session 3: **Life areas and values**, do one target activity
4. Session 4: **Valued activities**, do three target activities
5. Session 5: Review valued activities, schedule them
6. Session 6 (+P): Progress review, **contracts, problem-solving**
7. Session 7: New activity cycle, areas left to work on
8. Session 8 (+P): **Relapse prevention**
9. Review (+P): Review progress, review care plan

Note (+P) = with parent or carer input.

Clinician question: How should the eight sessions be spaced out?

We recommend that the first four sessions of Brief BA are completed within two weeks and that the next four sessions are weekly. Starting with sessions close together means that you and the young person can quickly build a relationship and can start to make changes as quickly as possible.

Sessions 1 + 2 = week 1, Sessions 3 + 4 = week 2

When scheduling your treatment sessions, it is important to check on holiday dates (both for yourself and the young person) as well as any times your service or setting might be closed, and plan around these. Sessions 1–6 are the most important to complete fairly close together, and it can sometimes help to space out the remaining sessions to give the young person more time to work on activities in between.

Finally, agree how the young person will cancel/re-arrange any sessions if needed, and what will help them remember the appointments. Remember, you want to make it as easy as possible for them to give Brief BA a try.

CHAPTER 3

Brief BA Sessions 1 and 2

Getting to Know the Young Person Better

Getting started and fitting it all in

There is a lot of ground to cover in Sessions 1 and 2. However, many of these are not discrete activities, so there is much overlap. For example, you will be building an alliance with the young person while you explain the Brief BA model to them and when you discuss their experiences and feelings, and negotiate how they would prefer you to involve their parents or carers. Sessions 1 and 2 also link closely together in terms of time. To make the most of Session 1, and to build hope and motivation to change, and to reduce the demands on memory, we recommend that you meet the young person twice in the same week. Ideally, Session 1 would take place on Monday or Tuesday and Session 2 on Thursday or Friday of the same week. This close scheduling is also helpful in planning the between-session work that you will ask the young person to do.

We also suggest you familiarize yourself with the session content well, and carefully plan how to manage your time in the first few sessions. The first session with both the young person and parent or carer has the added challenge of engaging two people (or possibly more, if more than one parent or carer attends) you may have never met. While we recommend that most sessions are no longer than an hour (to keep them focused and to minimize any burden on the young person), it might be helpful to allow slightly longer for the first session if you feel this would be useful.

Top tips for Sessions 1 and 2:

- ✓ The worksheets are designed to be used by *both the therapist and the young person* in the session
- ✓ The overwhelming feedback from young people has been that they want these worksheets to be in colour! You can download colour versions of the worksheets at https://library.jkp.com/redeem using the code TAUPAGE
- ✓ Ask the young person to bring their worksheets back to every session so they can be referred back to. Giving them a folder to keep their worksheets together can help with this
- ✓ Make sure you take a copy of any completed sections of worksheets
- ✓ Also provide parents or carers with a copy of their version of the worksheets at the same time (i.e. session by session)

✓ Think about the best way to share this if they are not at appointments (Email? Post? Asking the young person to pass them on?).

How to engage a depressed young person in Brief BA

■ **Young person:** 'I was somewhere I felt safe... I was listened to... I felt understood.'

The first and most important part of Brief BA is your relationship with the young person. Depression symptoms can make the most simple day-to-day activities hard work, and engaging in psychological therapy is an enormous demand. The young person's motivation for therapy can be low, and drop-out from treatment is common. No therapy will be effective if the person doesn't attend treatment sessions, so we emphasize engagement throughout Brief BA. This is particularly important at the start of your work where you'll be building the therapeutic relationship from scratch. Some of the ideas in Table 3.1 might be useful in building rapport and engaging a young person in Brief BA.

Table 3.1. How to engage a young person in Brief BA

Focus on the young person	Every young person is different; showing genuine curiosity about them will help you learn more and help them feel you really are interested in them
Show the young person you have kept them in mind	Keep a note of their friends', family's and pet's names, and refer back to things they've told you before (e.g. checking in about an exam they said was coming up)
Keep the young person central to the work	Make sure you don't get swayed too much by what parents or carers want (it can be easy to unintentionally align yourself with parents or carers when they are the dominant voices) Remember that the young person is the most important person in your work
Do your homework!	Ask about their interests or hobbies, do some research about these outside sessions, ask questions from them to learn more, ask for a lesson on a valued activity Use their interests and talents in therapy sessions whenever you can. For example, link 'healthy habits' to improving performance in sports they enjoy; redesign session worksheets with their artistic and creative input; explore favourite song lyrics relating to key Brief BA messages
Adapt Brief BA to fit the young person	Use electronic session worksheets if handwriting is challenging, and spider diagrams or cartoons of key messages Use their smartphone to set reminders, save photos of session worksheets, and make use of apps that can facilitate between-session work Make sessions shorter if they struggle to focus Make sessions active if they find it hard to sit still (e.g. go for a walk, do a valued activity together) Arrange the timing and frequency of sessions to fit their schedule
Offer your input outside sessions, and report back	Do your work between sessions just as you expect the young person to do between-session activities (e.g. contact their school to confirm their appointments and reduce their demands, research the pastoral support options in the college that they are due to start)
Be creative!!	Valued activation is the central component in Brief BA, so as long as you are helping the young person activate themselves and make positive changes in their behaviour, you can do this in many different ways

As a new therapist, you may find this engagement work a challenge, especially if you are used to working with younger children, with help-seeking and motivated adults, or with those whose primary difficulties are around anxiety. Bear this in mind when considering the beginning of your work with a depressed young person and speak with others who work with this client group to learn how they build rapport and engagement. You should also be mindful that their life might be very different from yours, and they may come from a cultural, racial, social, economic, sexual orientation or religious background that is unfamiliar to you and you may notice yourself drawing on stereotypes or limited knowledge. Having an open attitude and curiosity to learn about their *personal, unique experience* is essential.

Young people have consistently told us that having someone they trust to talk to has been a key helpful feature of Brief BA. Many will not have had any form of talking therapy or counselling before. This means that it's important to help 'set the scene' so they know what to expect from you and your Brief BA sessions together. Your relationship with them will be different from relationships they have with other adults. Most adults they know will be family members, or professionals – teachers, medical staff, sports coaches. You will be working with the young person in a collaborative way, and this might be completely new to them.

You should also remind them of confidentiality and the limits to this that apply in your particular setting. They need to be clear that the same rules apply every time you meet. You might say something like this:

- **Therapist:** 'Thank you for coming in again [name], I know how hard it can be to come to these sessions, especially at the start when we don't know each other very well. Today I'd like to spend some time getting to know you better and to understand how [depression/low mood/description that the young person uses] affects you. That'll help us work out how we might start to tackle this together using the Brief BA approach.'

Being collaborative

- **Young person:** 'It was a chilled-out approach, and almost like, friendly, you know? We worked together to figure things out, they didn't just tell me what to do.'

In Brief BA, the therapeutic alliance is built on collaboration. Brief BA is a joint effort, and there should be equal opportunity for the young person and the therapist to contribute. This joint effort can be hard because many young people see adults mainly in an authority role. Parents or carers and other adults also often view therapists as the 'expert', so it's important they get the idea of teamwork. This means that you may need to show the young person that they have a say in how their sessions run. It's helpful if you can demonstrate this to parents or carers as well.

There are some simple steps that can help encourage the young person to take more control of sessions:

- Ask them what they would like to talk about each session (and add it to the agenda)
- Check in with them before moving from one topic to another
- Ask them to describe how each Brief BA concept relates to them
- Ask them for ideas of between-session work
- Ask for feedback at the end of every Brief BA session, and make sure you use it; use feedback as a prompt for discussing your teamwork, and tell them that you need feedback from them to improve
- Empower them to be actively involved: they have control over the work.

Setting an agenda is one simple but powerful way to foster collaboration through Brief BA sessions. Agendas are used in all kinds of meetings, where the topics to be covered in the time allocated are discussed and agreed between attendees. There is then usually a process of checking in on this progress through agenda items. In psychological therapy, setting an agenda makes sure that time is well spent in every session, each person has an opportunity to suggest topics to cover, and important aspects are not missed because there has not been enough time.

How to set and use an agenda

1. Confirm how much time you have (be careful not to over-estimate this – if you have another session afterwards, you will need to leave time to write up your notes)
2. Make sure you factor in routine items that need to be covered at every session (e.g. completing and reviewing ROMs, agreeing between-session tasks, booking the next appointment)
3. Review what you can cover in the time available
4. Agree what you will prioritize, and allocate time for each item
5. During the session, check how you are doing with time management – are you sticking to time, do you need to move on, or do you need to adjust the agenda?
6. Highlight deviations from the agenda and discuss if you need to add any topic
7. Review the agenda at the end of the session and ask the young person for feedback – did you cover the most important things?

This process might feel unfamiliar to many young people, especially if you're in a setting where they are used to adults leading discussions and how time together is spent (e.g. in lessons at school). They may struggle to come up with items for the agenda in your early Brief BA sessions, but you can help them understand the purpose of this by introducing the idea from the start. This example script might be useful.

- **Therapist:** 'At the start of every time we meet we'll set an agenda. This is where we discuss what would be useful to cover in the session, think about what is most important, and how much time we should spend on each topic. This is to make sure that we're on the same page about how to make each session useful, and to ensure we use the time well. I'll keep an eye on this agenda during our sessions to make sure we leave enough time to cover the things we've agreed. I'll have some ideas for the agenda each week, but I also want to hear what you'd like us to talk about, so I'll ask you for your ideas each time too.'

Ongoing risk assessment

As we have already talked about, having suicidal thoughts is a symptom that many young people who have depression experience. A thorough risk assessment is essential during assessment, but it is also important to continue monitoring risk throughout your Brief BA sessions. This should be done in a way that uses information you have been told previously, checking in on what's changed since you last saw them rather than repeating everything from scratch (this can be understandably difficult to talk about, so make it as easy as possible for them to do so). You should include a risk check as a standard agenda item for every Brief BA session.

Psychoeducation: helping the young person understand about depression and the behavioural cycle of depression

- **Young person:** 'I understand myself more than I used to... I'm more self-aware of the traps I can easily fall into.'

Most adults (including many mental health professionals!) and young people know very little about depression in adolescents. They are usually not familiar with the full range of depression symptoms, or how they tend to present in adolescents. This can mean that symptoms of depression are not spotted, or that they are thought to mean something else altogether.

A common example is when parents and other adults see irritability in a young person as them being deliberately argumentative. This can mean that they respond with anger or irritability themselves, with the risk that they end up in an argument or at the least, feeling less close to the young person. If they knew that irritability is a core symptom of depression in adolescents, their reaction might be different and possibly more accepting and understanding.

Not understanding the symptoms of depression can also mean that young people, parents and therapists have unrealistic expectations of what the young person can manage. Often depression is marked by extreme fatigue and lack of energy, and this means that the young person simply cannot take part in many activities. Unrealistic expectations tend to lead to failure and disappointment – further exacerbating hopelessness and unhappiness. For these reasons, it's important to share information about depression in young people with the young person and, when possible, with their parent or carer. You will have explored the young person's individual depression symptoms in your assessment session, but it's helpful to review this and check if anything has changed (this also links to tracking progress – see later on in this section).

In the young person and parent worksheets for Session 1, the symptoms that are used to make a diagnosis of depression are highlighted. The young person and their parent or carer are encouraged to consider which of these symptoms the young person experiences. Because these do not capture the whole experience of depression, other common signs and problems are also included – sometimes, young people are surprised to see how varied the experience of depression can be. Seeing the symptoms written down together can be reassuring – if they are written down, it means that they are not completely alone and unique or 'weird', as other people must also feel the same way. Seeing the symptoms all written down can also feel overwhelming and increase their feelings of hopelessness. Be alert to this and note any change in the young person's behaviour that might indicate they feel differently. If you do notice such a change it can be very helpful to mention it, or to gently ask:

- **Therapist:** 'I noticed you seem a bit quiet since we looked at the different symptoms – what was that like for you?'

Some symptoms can be harder to spot and trickier to manage, and it can be helpful to identify these so you can work around them when planning changes. You might open a conversation about this with the young person in a number of different ways, for example:

- **Therapist:** 'As we talked about in the assessment, there are lots of different symptoms of depression and every young person has a different experience. It's important we recognize what symptoms are making life hard for you right now, and how we might work around these so they aren't barriers to you making the changes you want to make.'
- **Therapist:** 'You told me that making decisions has felt almost impossible since you started feeling down. This is a common symptom of depression, and might mean that choosing which valued activities to do might be tricky... If so, we can just try out activities one by one to see what gives you that feel-good factor.'
- **Therapist:** 'You've talked about how sleep is a big problem for you at the moment, which means you feel exhausted most of the time. Lot of depressed young people have sleep problems, which can get in the way of studying as well as focusing in Brief BA sessions. We can work around this by finding out more about your sleep and energy levels through the day, and keeping our Brief BA sessions short and booked in for times you feel more able to focus.' [Note: Many teenagers will prefer not to have an early morning appointment!]

The behavioural model of depression: explaining the Brief BA rationale

The rationale for Brief BA is simple – our aim is to make it as easy to understand and as uncomplicated as possible. The behavioural model highlights the link between rewards and mood. Thoughts and cognitions are not included, and there is no detailed or in-depth discussion about how and why the depression began, or about what early childhood experiences may have made a young person particularly vulnerable to depression.

The focus in Brief BA is on the 'here and now', so although it may be useful to understand possible triggers or causes of the young person's initial difficulties with depression, the intervention works on the maintenance cycle. This can be explained to young people and families as working on 'What is keeping depression going?' It is important to explain that we will be aiming to help the young person to make small behavioural changes on a daily basis, and that these that will help them feel better.

In Brief BA we try to streamline the message to the one key principle: Doing more of what matters helps boost your mood. Figure 3.1 below is used in the session and in the worksheets to help explain the Brief BA rationale and to work out how the link between rewards and mood works for the young person.

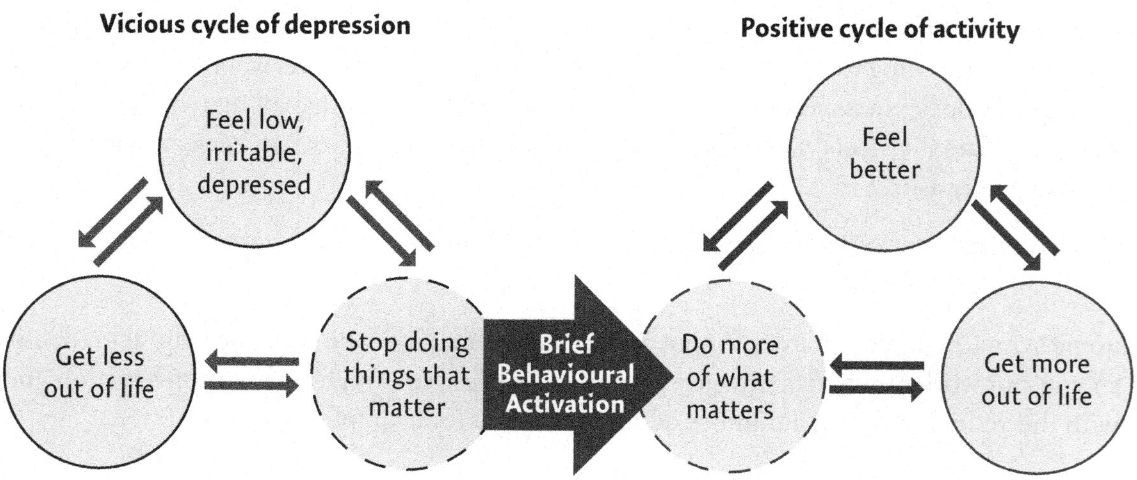

Figure 3.1. The Brief BA model

In the worksheets you will also see that we use two characters, Jayden and Sofia, to demonstrate how Brief BA works for different young people. Jayden and Sofia differ in important ways – they show how some young people with depression have very few activities (Jayden) and how others (Sofia) appear to be very busy but still experience very little reward. You can use Jayden and Sofia as examples throughout your Brief BA sessions. For example, in Session 1 you could use one or other (or both) characters to draw how the Brief BA model works for them.

We'd encourage you to draw the Brief BA model with the young person, using their own experience to fill in each part of the diagram. You can do this on a piece of paper, or for greater effect, on a whiteboard or flipchart. What's most important is to use their own words and examples to make the cycle real and meaningful for them. For example: 'When I started *feeling down* after splitting up with my girlfriend, I stopped spending as much time with my friends after school – this means *I just sit in my room* and *feel sad and lonely*.' It is important to consider how specific depression symptoms might be fuelling this vicious cycle of depression. For example, if someone has lost interest or pleasure in usually enjoyable activities (anhedonia), it's completely normal to have less enthusiasm for doing these things. Similarly, concentration problems can make sitting through a film with friends much harder than it used to be.

When the therapist and young person have filled in the cycle using the young person's own examples and words, they move across to the positive cycle. It is important for the therapist to explain the positive cycle of activity in a simple but non-patronizing way. For example, we've found the following ways of explaining it useful:

- **Therapist:** 'By understanding what matters to you, we can work together to figure out activities that will give you that sense of reward. When you do these activities, that reward boosts your mood, which makes it easier to do more activities to give you more reward, so it kick-starts the positive cycle of activity.'
- **Therapist:** 'It's important to recognize that it's not easy to just "do more of what matters", otherwise you would have already done it. There are lots of reasons why this can be tough, especially when the symptoms of depression get in the way. It also doesn't mean that things will change overnight – it's taken a while for the cycle of depression to build up, so it will take a while for us to reverse it. That's why we're going to work together on this, as a team – with my help, and help from [parents or carers, other important adults] together we'll come up with a step-by-step plan that you can manage and that feels achievable.'

Top tips for explaining the Brief BA rationale:

- ✓ To explain the Brief BA model clearly and well you need to genuinely believe it! To get used to explaining the model we recommend that all Brief BA therapists use self-practice to learn how it feels to complete the worksheets and use the techniques of Brief BA themselves (see 'Brief BA self-practice' in Chapter 2)
- ✓ If possible, use a time in your own life when you felt down and got less reward. We also recommend you role-play to practise explaining the Brief BA model to someone. This can be with a colleague, your supervisor or a trainer. Swap places and make sure you give each other feedback about how the explanation came across
- ✓ Some other things that might be useful include:

- Use pen and paper, a whiteboard or chalkboard to draw out the cycle
- Acknowledge that it is hard to get out of a vicious cycle, and you can feel trapped
- Use the young person's own words for their experience (e.g. how do they describe their depression?)
- Clarify that it's about increasing meaningful activities (linked to what matters to them), not just about enjoyment or fun
- Link back to information you already have about their experience, so they feel understood and can see how this relates to them personally
- Briefly mention the evidence behind Brief BA: this increases confidence that such a simple sounding treatment actually works
- Emphasize that the *young person* will decide what matters, and the activities relating to this (it helps to state this explicitly in front of parents or carers from the start)
- Be mindful of any constraints they might be limited by (e.g. physical disability or illness, financial or logistical challenges), and be realistic about ways round this.

Clinician question: But won't it sound patronizing to just tell young people 'Do more'?

Yes, and that's not the message of Brief BA!

- It is important that you are very clear, right from the start, that Brief BA is not just about doing *more*; Brief BA is about doing *more of what matters*
- It is also important to highlight that Brief BA is about doing more of what matters *to them* (i.e. not what is important to other people)
- In Session 3, you will spend time with the young person identifying their values – this is how you and they work out *what matters to them*
- Emphasize the importance of values, and how taking this approach is likely to be different from ideas they've tried. Provide lots of empathy and validation of their experience, and any attempts they've made to change in the past. If it was easy to change they'd already have done it and wouldn't be seeing you
- Be clear with parents or carers so they don't provide an unhelpful message at home.

Therapist: 'I think keeping it simple and positive is what I found to be the most helpful things to make Brief BA successful...focusing on that positive reinforcement, Brief BA, it's all about that. So if a young person has come in and not done something but they had done another thing, just really focusing on the positives and then also helping them problem-solve and break down that activity into smaller steps.'

Engaging and working with parents and carers

Where possible, we always try to involve the young person's parents or carers in treatment. We do this for a number of practical reasons. In many cases it is the parent of the young person who has sought out treatment and encouraged their son or daughter to come to the sessions. As parents, they experience worry and distress watching their son or daughter being unhappy and not able to fully enjoy life. They almost always want to help their child, but they very often do not know how to do this.

Another important reason to involve parents in treatment is to support young people who are at risk of self-harm or suicide. If important information needs to be shared in order to keep the young person safe, this is much easier for the therapist, the young person and the parent if there is already an established relationship and communication route with parents.

In addition to providing general support and encouragement and keeping their son or daughter safe, parents can help the young person access more positive reinforcement and reward. Often parents and carers have access to resources and rewards. Rewards do not need to involve money. They can be tangible rewards, for example a lift to see a friend, a favourite meal or company on a walk with the dog. They can also be intangible – a hug, a smile, an encouraging word and praise.

There can also be challenges with involving parents or carers in Brief BA. Parents and carers can make rewards harder to access or more difficult, and can actively reduce rewards and therefore increase the young person's feeling of depression. In these cases it is even more important to work with them, to help them understand the Brief BA rationale, explore any concerns they may have, and consider how Brief BA can work within their individual family and house rules. Other times, there may be practical barriers to involving parents, for example if English is not their first language, they have a disability or health condition that makes travel difficult, or they have other care commitments that prevent them from attending appointments. It is important that these issues do not disadvantage the young person or family from accessing the same level of support as other families, so you should work within your specific team and service to overcome such barriers. For example, use of in-person or phone interpreters is usually possible with advance planning, and many services have access to these professional services.

Sometimes it is not possible to work with parents and carers. However, when we do, the feedback we get is very positive.

- **Young person:** 'I liked having the chance to talk with and without mum, and to talk to someone else.'

- **Parent:** 'I really valued and appreciated the contact and feedback after the initial assessment. It was reassuring and the email updates and sheets were also helpful.'

We suggest involving parents or carers in Brief BA in the following ways:

- Invite parents or carers in to some part of Brief BA sessions, particularly at the beginning and final sessions
- Give parents their own copy of the Brief BA worksheets
- Make sure that parents understand the Brief BA model of depression and how treatment will work – psychoeducation for parents
- Make sure they understand how their child's symptoms of depression are affecting them
- Have catch-up phone calls if they are unable to attend sessions
- Identify and then problem-solve any barriers parents may present for the young person making progress in Brief BA
- Share information with parents as agreed with the young person (including risk).

Using parents or carers to increase rewards for the young person

We encourage young people to 'Do more of what matters' so that they receive more rewards (positive reinforcement). Increasing positive reinforcement is a central component of Brief BA. Given how hard it can be to make changes (i.e. to 'Do more of what matters') while fighting against depression symptoms, young people need as much help as they can get. Parents or carers and other important adults are in a key role to offer reinforcement for any attempt the young person makes at non-depressed behaviour. However, depressed young people can be hard to be around and engage with, and some parents can struggle to see the effort that is needed by the young person to make even small changes. That's why it can be useful to get them involved at the start of Brief BA, to help explain the rationale and to understand how they can best help. Parents are kept involved throughout Brief BA, but it's especially important to get them on board at the start.

Clinician question: How should I involve parents or carers in Brief BA?

We typically suggest that parents or carers are invited to attend part of Sessions 1, 6 and 8. It is important for the therapist to take into account the preferences of the young person when deciding when to include parents and for how long. When you invite parents or carers into the session, have a clear plan about how you will involve them. Consider ways of supporting the young person in the sessions where their parents are present (e.g. where you sit, elicit the young person's views and opinions, and ensure a balance between their own and their parents' input).

Top tip: If you have any contact with adults (parents, carers, school staff, other professionals involved in their care) when the young person is not present, always tell the young person about this so they do not feel you are going behind their back. Young people have told us how important this is and how it can affect the trust they have with you in the therapy room.

Involving other adults

The rules of consent and confidentiality (that are specific to your context) will apply to all information sharing. Although it is important to be careful about what is shared and with whom, it is helpful for Brief BA therapists to emphasize the benefits of joining up support when starting Brief BA sessions.

Some suggestions of who to link up with are given below. This is not an exhaustive list and we would encourage you to ask the young person 'Who else might be able to help support you when we're doing Brief BA work?' Examples include:

- School or college staff (informing them about absences for attendance at Brief BA sessions, sharing information to facilitate additional support at school, considering extenuating circumstances for exams, finding a school- or college-based coach who can help keep progress going after Brief BA has ended)
- Family doctor (to share risk and treatment information, check in on any physical health conditions or symptoms that may relate to a physical health need)
- All caregivers, even if the young person is not living with them (often these caregivers can get left out of therapy, so are particularly important to remember)
- Medical teams managing chronic or debilitating conditions

- Any other professionals involved with the young person (e.g. youth offending or justice system, social care etc.)
- Other important adults who can play a supportive, reinforcing role (e.g. close family friend, stepmum, godparent, relatives the young person feels are particularly helpful).

Table 3.2. Challenges of involving others and potential solutions

Challenge	Potential solutions
Young person does not want parents or carers involved	Discuss how to involve parents or carers without sharing personal details (e.g. providing handouts, having general conversations about Brief BA content without the specifics relating to the young person) Agree what can or can't be shared; explore the reasons behind this and problem-solve if there are any barriers that can be easily overcome Find out if there are other important adults who could be involved instead of parents or carers (e.g. aunt, grandfather, older adult sibling, stepparent, school pastoral lead, college tutor) Review involvement of others regularly as initial reluctance could reduce through therapy
Parents or carers do not appear motivated to be involved	Ask them to come to a session Emphasize that this is a central part of treatment Discuss ways to make this as feasible as possible (e.g. if childcare or work commitments make coming to sessions difficult, arrange a phone call or email updates)
Conflict between young person and parent or carer	Use Brief BA contracts and problem-solving to explore this with the young person and adult(s) Emphasize the importance of improving relationships as central to the young person's recovery Be mindful that in cases of serious, escalating conflict, there may be safeguarding issues – bring any concerns to supervision
Parent or carer has own mental health problems that make it hard for them to support the young person	Encourage parent or carer to seek help for their own mental health Signpost to relevant services and support for adults Encourage parent or carer to use Brief BA principles as a family (e.g. 'Doing more of what matters', engaging in shared valued activities)
Parent or carer does not complete agreed actions between sessions	Use problem-solving strategies Consider how to make this easier for parents or carers (e.g. increased communication about this, getting young person to check in on potential actions for parents or carers before agreeing them) Explore who else might be able to help the young person between sessions (e.g. other relative, older sibling, school)

Tracking progress in Brief BA with Routine Outcome Measures (ROMs)

Young person: 'I liked that I could track my progress and see my mood slowly go up each week; it was a subtle change but in the right direction.'

Every time we meet a young person we want to know how they are doing. In Brief BA we use Routine Outcome Measures (ROMs) as a way of checking in every week. Typically, in the UK at least, therapists will use ROMs to quickly assess the young person's key symptoms, self-harm or suicidal thoughts or behaviours, their general wellbeing and functioning, and how the session has been for the young person.

You may already work in a service that uses ROMs, and more and more services are moving in this direction. We are advocates of using ROMs and there are many reasons for this. Clinically it makes sense because it means that the young person and therapist are continually checking in on how therapy is going, and the level of current difficulties the young person is experiencing. By including the parent report where possible, it also allows the therapist to identify similarities and differences in the young person and their parents' views. In addition, because we also use ROMs to assess risk at every session, any increase in risk will be noticed and can be dealt with immediately. ROMs provide a standard way to review all the young people you are working with, and this is very useful as a way of summarizing your work and highlighting individual young people who it would be useful to discuss in supervision. Finally, there is some evidence that using ROMs is associated with better treatment outcomes. We will discuss the evidence for this in Part 3 of the manual.

Tracking progress should therefore be part of every Brief BA session, and the reasons for doing this should be clearly explained to both the young person and parents or carers. While many people are used to completing questionnaires for an assessment, completing session-by-session measures is often less familiar, so the rationale for this should be given. An example of how this might be introduced is given below.

Therapist: 'In Brief BA, it's important we keep checking in on how you're finding the sessions, and how you are doing generally to see if Brief BA is helping. By doing this every time we meet, we can make sure we catch any problems early on and try to problem-solve them by doing things differently. It also helps me get to know you better, to see what things are difficult for you each week and where things might start to change more quickly. It also means that I can keep an eye on whether I need to ask my supervisor for advice.'

Any questionnaires you ask young people and/or parents or carers to complete must always be explained fully before you ask them to fill them in (so you need to make sure you really understand what each questionnaire is asking, and why!), and you should always discuss the scores and their meaning every time a questionnaire has been completed.

Key Routine Outcome Measures for use in Brief BA

Your service may already have a set of measures used by everyone – obviously you should continue to use these. In our practice, we use the following measures at every session:

- Revised Child Anxiety and Depression Scale (RCADS; Chorpita *et al.* 2000). We use the ten-item depression subscale and add an extra item to ask about suicidal thoughts ('I have thought about killing myself')
- Outcome Rating Scale (ORS; Miller and Duncan 2000)
- Session Rating Scale (SRS; Duncan *et al.* 2003).

Many measures are freely available (including all versions of the RCADS) and can be downloaded from the Child Outcomes Research Consortium (CORC) website.[1] Further information on the licence agreements for the ORS, SRS and associated scales (e.g. CORS) can be found on this website, along with lots of useful information about a wide variety of ROMs, and on measuring change in Child and Adolescent Mental Health services.

1 www.corc.uk.net

Table 3.3. Routine outcome measures used in Child and Adolescent Mental Health services

Brief name	Full name	Purpose	Clinical thresholds?
RCADS	Revised Child Anxiety and Depression Scale	Total scores + subscales for depression and anxiety disorders Used at start and end of treatment	Yes (for specific age, gender, informant)
RCADS-Dep	RCADS Depression Subscale + Risk Q	Brief depression measure, additional risk Q added ('I've thought of killing myself') Used at every session	Yes (for specific age, gender, informant)
ORS	Outcome Rating Scale	Functioning in four areas: individual, interpersonal, social, overall Used at every session	Yes (28)
GBO	Goal-based outcomes	Client identified goals for treatment Used at every session	No (0–10 rating)
SRS	Session Rating Scale	Brief measure of therapeutic alliance Used at every session	No, but a score below 36 should always be discussed

It is important that any questionnaires you use should be suitable for the person you're asking to complete them. The above measures are suitable for young people aged 11–18 and are relatively brief so do not take too much time or effort to complete. They are also relatively simple to interpret. Make sure you are using ROMs that are appropriate, and make adaptations if needed. This might include reading questions for the young person, helping them to understand what specific words mean and making sure they don't miss out questions.

❓ Clinician question: How do I use the questionnaires (ROMs) in a clinically meaningful way?

- Score these up as soon as possible, in session if you can
- Use a visual depiction of the ROMs by plotting scores on a graph across sessions. Include the young person's and parent's or carer's scores on different lines
- For ROMs with clinical thresholds, keep a note of these and identify them on your graphs (remember that these may be different scores for different ages or gender and self or parent report)
- Always discuss ROMs if you have asked for them to be completed
- Always ask for feedback at the end of every session to see if there is anything (big or small) that the young person would like to do differently. If a young person struggles to give you suggestions, ask what they liked, to find out what you should keep doing
- Ask the young person and parent or carer for feedback on what they think the scores reflect. Be clear about how gathering this information adds to the other sources of information you have (verbal report, therapist's view)
- Discuss ROMs in supervision. No change in ROMs after three sessions or a steep deterioration between sessions should always be taken to supervision. This may indicate poor engagement with Brief BA, difficulties in the therapeutic relationship or external factors that need addressing in order for young person to make progress.

Identifying goals for treatment

Goals should be identified at the start of Brief BA, to understand what the young person wants to work on through the treatment. Goal-based outcomes (GBOs) are different from symptom or functioning measures, as they measure progress towards a self-identified target the young person wants to achieve, that is, where and what they want to aim for. Ideally, goals should be positively framed, and a young person may need help to see how their initial ambitions to stop or reduce certain thoughts ('I want to stop hating myself so much'), feelings ('I want to feel less depressed') or behaviours ('I want to argue less with mum and dad') could be reframed towards a positive target. This helps set the positive stance that runs throughout the whole of Brief BA, and also means that progress is seen as steps forward towards a positive target that can be easier to recognize than reductions of negative aspects.

Therapist: 'To understand what to focus on in our work together, it's helpful to identify some goals. If our Brief BA sessions were helpful, by the end of our time working together, what would you like to have changed? Where would you want to be that is different from where you are now?'

Goals should be as *SMART* as possible:

- ***S****pecific:* What exactly is it that the young person wants to achieve?
- ***M****easurable:* How will you and they know when they have made progress towards it? What would they be doing if they got to a 5, 8, 10?
- **A***chievable:* What is going to be possible to aim for right now? Don't aim too high
- ***R****ealistic and* ***R****elevant:* Is this feasible with the resources available? Will it really make a difference if this thing changed?
- ***T****ime-specific:* What is the time period for the young person to achieve this goal? When do they want to achieve it? In the next month? By the end of Brief BA? By the end of this year?

Sometimes goals are identified at the end of assessments and, if so, these should be reviewed at the start of Brief BA and amended as necessary. Some goals may be beyond the scope of Brief BA while others may be particularly relevant. Usually, behaviourally oriented goals align especially well with the Brief BA model. Goals that focus on emotions can often be made more measurable by considering the associated behaviours. If the young person identifies a feeling, try asking, 'How would you know you were feeling that way?' and, 'What would you be doing that you are not doing now?' For example, 'Feel happier' can be made SMARTer by considering how others would notice that in the young person and what would be observable, such as 'Going out with my friends twice a week during school term time'.

The most helpful goals in Brief BA will be different for every young person, and the most important element is that they are identified by them. Some examples of goals young people have identified and worked on through Brief BA are given below:

- Complete eight hours of revision a week: by the end of Brief BA
- Be able to have a conversation with a teacher I don't usually speak to: by the end of this term
- Do one thing I enjoy each day: by two weeks' time

- Get into make-up again (e.g. practising on self) and be able to do this: in a couple of weeks
- Spend one hour each day on an activity relating to only me: by the end of Brief BA
- Eat with my family twice a week: by Diwali
- Walk the dog before school once a week and once a day on weekends: by half-term
- Join a team outside school that will be challenging and involve being more active: by one month from now
- Meet up with friends once a week: by the end of the month
- Do some art every day (including doodling): within two weeks
- Do homework the day I get it: within one month
- Get my grades back up to pass or above: in one month.

Goals should be written down and rated for current progress (where 10 = fully achieved and 0 = not yet started towards this goal). How regularly you check in on progress towards goals should be agreed with the young person, but this should be done at least every few sessions to monitor how Brief BA is working on the issues most relevant to the young person.

Activity monitoring

Young person: 'When I recorded what I was doing and wrote it down, I could see if what I was doing was actually productive and if it actually made me feel any better...so then it would be like "Oh, if this isn't making me feel better is there's anything else that I could replace that with?"'

Activity monitoring is the first kind of *between*-session work that we ask young people to do in Brief BA. To set this up properly, it's essential that you first go through this together *in* the session.

Activity monitoring is incredibly helpful for the Brief BA therapist, because:

- It's a quick, easy way to see how a young person is spending their time
- It can provide rich information about their life outside the therapy room
- Agreeing the most suitable way for them to complete this first homework task will give you ideas of how they might find it easiest to engage in Brief BA
- It helps emphasize the importance of behaviour and the link between activities and mood.

Framing the activity log as a 'getting to know you' tool can help young people understand that you are genuinely interested in how they spend their days, in order to work together to identify changes they want to and feel able to make.

Therapist: 'To start with, I'd like to get to know you better so we can make Brief BA work for you. We also need to figure out how you're spending your time at the moment, to see where you might want to make changes.'

Activity monitoring is a great tool for both of these things:

- **Therapist:** 'By noting down what you've been doing between our sessions and then us reviewing this when we meet, I'll find out much more about you than I'd be able to just by asking you questions. Having a record also helps us both to see patterns and detail in your life that could give us clues about easy places to start.'
- **Therapist:** 'How many days you keep the record, how often and how much detail you record is completely flexible, and we can talk about ways this can work to make sure this feels manageable for you.'

At this point, it's useful to emphasize one of the key mottos of Brief BA: *No activity is no activity.* What we are trying to get across here is that everyone has behaviour they can record. Every minute of the day we are doing something, whether that's a clearly defined leisure activity we would describe to others (e.g. watching a film), a more routine daily task (e.g. having a shower) or behaviours we often disregard as activities (e.g. sleeping, daydreaming).

Flexibility with activity monitoring

There are lots of ways that a young person can record their daily activities. The most simple is a paper form showing each day, and breaking this down into hours of the day. The person recording their activities simply writes down what they were doing throughout the day, so the activity record is really a detailed kind of diary. The same form can also be completed digitally, on a computer or phone diary, or on one of many available phone apps. The easiest way to decide how a young person should monitor their activity is to *ask them what will work best for them.* They will have a good idea of what feels manageable and fits into their everyday life.

There is a blank activity log worksheet that you can fill in together available to download at https://library.jkp.com/redeem using the code TAUPAGE. There are also examples of activity monitoring forms completed by Jayden and Sofia. You will notice that Sofia's is more detailed than Jayden's – this is important, to show the young person that they have some choice in how much information to record and how much detail to include. You can also invite them to adapt or enhance the activity monitoring worksheets to suit themselves.

Achievement, Closeness, Enjoyment and Importance ratings

In addition to recording the activities that the young person does each day, we ask them to record their ratings of Achievement, Closeness, Enjoyment (ACE) and Importance (I).[2] ACE-I recording helps to capture the range of rewards that young people experience from their activities:

Achievement – Young people who are depressed often find that academic work is extremely difficult and feel that they are failing. However, they can often recognize achievement when they manage to attend a lesson, complete a homework assignment or get to school on time. Other daily chores or tasks can also give some level of achievement (e.g. tidying their room, cleaning out their pet's cage).

Closeness – Adolescence is a time when friendships, romantic or family relationships can be especially important, so it's helpful to identify activities that bring a sense of closeness (and those

2 We use the ACE recording from www.getselfhelp.co.uk (developed by and with kind permission from Carol Vivyan).

that don't). Some activities without any physical proximity to others may still create this sense of closeness (e.g. looking at photos from a special family event, remembering a loved one on an anniversary), while it is also possible to feel alone even when you're with others. Closeness can also be felt through companionship with animals, and spiritual closeness.

Enjoyment – This is pretty straightforward; was the activity to some degree fun? Because enjoyment and pleasure is often absent or very rare when young people are depressed, any time we can notice and identify enjoyment (even if brief or at a low level) is worthwhile.

Importance – Importance ratings help draw the focus onto the value of activities from the first session of Brief BA. It is important to emphasize that this refers to whether the activity is important to them; it does not refer to how important the activity is to other people. This rating will give you an instant idea about valued and non-valued activities in their lives currently, and help to start the conversation about what matters to them.

Often, young people will identify very few important activities; this is a useful prompt for asking what they would prefer to have been doing or what is missing.

There can sometimes be grey areas with this. For example, some young people are clear that school is important to them (or at least some of the lessons that they feel matter to them and their future). Others are clear that school is not something that matters to them, and that they go only under duress. Another young person might acknowledge that while school is not important to them personally, their parents and school staff believe it is, and attending means that they do not get in trouble. Therefore, it is important to them for this reason. There is no right or wrong here, and it's important you emphasize to the young person that it's about what really matters to them (and what doesn't) rather than what they think they should say or other people would think. This is an important reason why we recommend completing the activity log together before setting it for homework. This way you can make sure that the young person fully understands the task.

Mood ratings in activity monitoring

Linking activities to mood is key when activity monitoring. This can be done by giving an overall mood rating for each day, or if the young person feels their mood fluctuates a lot, they can rate it at different points of the day (e.g. after each activity, every few hours, etc.).

Top tips: Keep in mind these points when explaining activity monitoring to the young person:

- ✓ This is a way to get to know the young person better, by learning about what they do every day
- ✓ Allocate sufficient time in session to explain the rationale and go through an example fully
- ✓ Adapt activity monitoring to the young person (personalize frequency, duration, detail and ratings as well as method of recording)
- ✓ Be flexible. Work to their strengths (e.g. computer skills, use of mobile-based calendar or task lists)
- ✓ Be open about the need for this to work for them, and agree the level of detail that is realistic
- ✓ Check their understanding and level of engagement before setting the homework task

✓ Encourage any effort and set expectations low; use parental support or facilitation of the task if the young person finds this acceptable

✓ Don't ask for too much. It's unrealistic for most depressed young people to complete an activity log every day for a week. It's helpful to collect information about a school or work day compared to a leisure day, if they are able to

✓ Discuss together how many days (and which days) the young person feels able to record, and agree how they will remember to do it on those days

✓ Think about what the young person might want to record (e.g. activities, meals, sleep, exercise)

✓ If a young person is self-harming, ask them to record this in the same way as they would with any other activity

✓ Be aware that this process can be confronting for some young people (seeing their depressed life in black and white on paper). Discuss how to use this as a step for positive change

✓ Link the activity monitoring back to the key rationale in Brief BA: small changes can make a big difference, but we need the detail to find where these small changes could happen.

Reviewing the activity log

Reviewing an activity log is a key task in Session 2. It is *essential* that having given the young person an important task to do between sessions, you take the time to carefully discuss their activity log with them and use it to get to know them better. Imagine if someone asked you to do some extra work in your own time, told you how important this was and explained the reasons why, you put that time and effort into doing it, and then they never mentioned it again!

■ **Young person:** 'It helped me realize what I do day-to-day is not what I enjoy doing, and encouraged me to do more of what I enjoy.'

❓ **Clinician question:** How do I review the activity log with the young person?

First of all, make sure that you praise them for doing the activity log and bringing it back to the session. Use any material they bring back, however minimal.

The easiest way to make sure you've fully understood the young person's activity log is to ask them to talk you through it. You could then ask clarification questions as you go, such as:

- What does [activity] exactly look like?
- Where were you when you did [activity]?
- Was anyone with you when you did [activity]? [If so] Who?
- [If using general term like 'friend', 'brother', 'teacher'] Which friend/brother/teacher?
- [If using general statement like 'lessons'] What lessons were they? What happens before/between/after lessons?
- [If using general statement like 'Go to...'] How do you get there? How long does it take?

- [If a number of activities have been grouped together, e.g. 'chilled after college, made dinner, watched TV'] Which bit of that activity gave you those ratings? Would you give different ratings for the individual things you did?
- What was it about [activity] that meant you rated it that way?
- What would have been a higher rated activity or how might this activity rate higher?

As well as making sure that you take the activity log seriously and value their efforts to complete the task between sessions, it also gives you an opportunity to develop a much more detailed understanding of the young person's daily life. However, this may not be immediately obvious, and you may need to use information in the activity log to prompt further discussion and clarification. Table 3.4 illustrates how unpacking a simple behavioural record can mean very different things for two different young people.

Table 3.4: Clarifying how the same activity log entry might mean very different things

Activity log entry	
'Get ready for school'	
What this actually involves:	
Sasha	Amy
Wake up, throw some clothes on, grab coat, leave house	Wake up, wake up sister, shower, style hair, do make-up, iron uniform, make breakfast for myself and sister, eat breakfast, wash up bowls, tidy kitchen, finish History homework, pack bag, get coat, leave house

Useful questions to ask in an activity log review include:

- What was it like filling it in?
- What did you notice?
- What stood out to you?
- Is there anything missing that might be on here from a different day, or that you wish was on here?
- What have you taken away from looking at how you spend your time?
- Has it made you think differently about how you spend your time?
- How can we make sure this activity log feels manageable to complete again?
- Would it be useful to get any help from [relevant adults] to do this?

❓ **Clinician question:** What would the ideal activity log look like?

There is no ideal! Everyone is different, but generally speaking, an activity log showing a range of activities that give some high ACE ratings and are also rated as Important to the young person is a very good sign. This indicates that they are likely to be experiencing diverse and stable sources of positive reinforcement in their daily life. Often these activities can be quite brief, but the fact they are interspersed around less valued activities suggests the young person is 'topping up' their reward tank regularly.

Clinician question: What should I do if a young person is keen to make changes from our initial discussion in Session 1?

This is great! If they have had information about the Brief BA rationale, and this fits with how they want to move forwards, they might already have some idea of how they want to spend their time differently.

- Be clear that this is okay. Encourage and support this, and praise their motivation
- Ask them to record this on their activity log (or another way of logging it that is acceptable to them), and make sure you discuss in the next session: 'Which activities did you try to do more/less of?'

Clinician question: What do I do if a young person doesn't complete the activity log?

First of all, don't worry – this is very common. It doesn't mean that you are a bad therapist or that the young person cannot benefit from Brief BA. For a depressed young person, completing the activity log on their own between sessions requires a lot of organization, motivation and energy. Often they simply cannot overcome these problems. It is important to use this situation as an opportunity to explore what would work better for them. Table 3.5 outlines some ways to move forward collaboratively.

Table 3.5. What to do and what not to do if a young person has not completed their activity log homework

DO NOT	DO
Tell them off or act as if you are disappointed in them	Identify things that got in the way of completing the activity log, e.g.: • Lack of explanation from you • Overly high expectations by you • Not enough time • Too difficult • Forgetting
Think that this means Brief BA won't work	Use problem-solving to identify what the young person could do to overcome barriers
Give up hope!	Emphasize other ways that the young person could complete the activity log and be creative
Avoid thinking/talking about this	Praise any attempts they made to complete the activity log
	Complete the activity log with them in the session to show them how important it is to collect this information (and what you will do with it)
	Discuss in supervision and consider how you might do it differently next time

CHAPTER 4

Brief BA Session 3

What Matters to the Young Person?

What is important to young people?

■ **Young person:** 'It helped me think about how certain things I do actually improve my mood because they're important to me, so I want to do more of them...and other things are like "Oh, I don't actually need to do that, that doesn't really do anything for me."'

Young people typically have limited autonomy and control over their everyday lives, with certain activities mandated (such as school, college or training) and others prohibited (such as driving, voting or drinking before a certain age). Some of these constraints may be there for very good reasons, while others might feel more arbitrary. As an adult, it's easy to forget how much control we have over our lives now compared to our younger years – we've got used to it!

Given the constraints that are imposed on young people, it's especially important to understand what the individual young person finds important. Depending on their view, they may be engaged in activities that are personally meaningful and rewarding for them (e.g. doing well at school is important to them, so attending is not a chore), or they may find themselves stuck with activities that offer little, if any, personal reward.

It's easy to assume all young people will have similar values and place importance on certain things. In fact, we've heard a staggering range and diversity of values from the young people we've worked with, both clinically and in a research setting. Table 4.1 illustrates a small selection of values identified by young people we have worked with. Therapists, too, have a range of different values. Your own values, as well as stereotypes and societal norms, will influence your expectations as a Brief BA therapist. This means that it is important to be aware of them so that you know how they affect you at work, as well as elsewhere. It also means that it is vital to maintain a curious and open approach when exploring values with a young person – as long as their values aren't damaging or dangerous (which, in our experience, is hardly ever the case). There is no right or wrong answer here.

Table 4.1. Values held by young people

Example values from our Brief BA clients		
Me	**Things that matter**	**People who matter**
Eat healthily	Be organized	Spend time with mum
Art	Pass my exams	Help others

cont.

Example values from our Brief BA clients		
Me	**Things that matter**	**People who matter**
Chill out	Church	Keep in touch
Make time for me	Volunteering	Be a caring friend
Exercise	Get a job	Be positive with others
Get enough sleep	Focus on tasks	Help my family out
Rugby	Be tidy	Catch up with my sister
Guitar	Human rights	Be a good friend
Meditate	Learn about journalism	Help grandparents
Get out of the house	Be productive	Be a good listener
Skateboarding	Use time efficiently	Connect with friends
Do a variety of activities	Everything German	Make time for my boyfriend

Helping a young person identify their values

Your conversation about values may well be the first time a young person has been asked about what's important to them. Although it may feel like a challenging topic to discuss in therapy (especially with a depressed young person), our experience shows that young people (11- to 18-year-olds, both with and without depression symptoms) are able to identify personally important values using the life areas and values worksheet from Brief BA. In Table 4.1, the values are arranged in three categories or life areas: 'Me' (individual values about themselves), 'Things that matter' (general aspects of how they want to live their lives) and 'People who matter' (interpersonal values). These life areas are used in the worksheets to help young people think about what matters *to them*. You will also find examples from Sofia and Jayden to show young people concrete examples of what we mean when we talk about their values (i.e. what matters to them) in Part 4.

Sometimes it might be hard to talk about their values, especially if they are far removed from how a young person is living at the moment, or the young person is concerned about how you will view their values. They might expect you to disapprove or disagree with their values. This is where your relationship building throughout Brief BA will help – young people are much more likely to open up if they feel they can trust you.

When exploring values with the young person using the life areas and values worksheet, they don't need to identify a value in every box, and each box can have more than one value in them. There are also blank boxes at the bottom for values that don't quite fit under any of the suggested headings (these are there as prompts, not requirements!).

Often hobbies can be an easy way to start, as usually young people are able to tell you some kind of leisure activity they find at least somewhat enjoyable or important to them. You will also have collected a wealth of information from assessment, session discussion and activity monitoring that can help guide possible ideas for you to suggest if a young person is struggling. For example, you might remember things they enjoy or did enjoy from your questions around the symptom of anhedonia in the assessment session.

There are also some 'healthy habits' that can be helpful to suggest working on if a young person is hesitant to know where to start, especially if their everyday routines are significantly disrupted. Maintaining a regular sleep/wake cycle, mealtimes and activity levels while limiting use of substances (including sugar, nicotine and alcohol) and screen time (from computers, phones, tablets, etc.) is generally good for everyone's wellbeing. However, be careful not to put too much emphasis on these aspects if a young person has not voiced a desire to work on them. While these aspects of routine can generally be helpful for emotional wellbeing, they are already likely to have had similar messages from other adults, and may have reasons for not pursuing them. Often a young person will identify some healthy habits as part of their individual values, but these are specific to what is important to them (e.g. getting a good night's sleep, eating more fruit and veg).

Top tip: Remember that it can take some time for us to articulate what matters to us. Give them plenty of space and pace your questioning to make sure you don't rush to fill any silences where the young person is just thinking. If you haven't tried completing your own life areas and values worksheet, do it now – you'll have a much better understanding of what this is like for your clients.

Some values may indicate areas of conflict between current behaviour and views on how the young person wants to live (e.g. current substance use conflicts with 'Looking after myself' value), so can be a way in to discuss unhelpful behaviours. It is important to recognize that a young person's values may not be the same as those of their therapist, parent(s) or carer(s), sibling(s) or peers. However, valued activities should be encouraged in all instances except where there are direct negative consequences or they are known to be harmful (e.g. drug taking, going directly against family rules). Any concern over such values should be taken to supervision.

Clinician question: Won't a young person just tell me values or activities they think I want to hear?

This is less common than you think if you have set up the therapeutic relationship well! It's critical that you emphasize the importance of what is important to them, not anybody else, and that's what you want to learn about. Some generic values (e.g. 'be a good friend') are likely to apply to most young people. The assessment details, content of early sessions and the activity log will give you ideas about possible values for the young person – highlighting these things they've already told you may encourage them to think more personally.

The difference between goals, activities and values

Some therapists can get caught up trying to separate out whether what the young person identifies fits best under a value, or if it is better considered as an activity, or possibly even a goal. If a young person identifies a value you feel may be more of a specific activity (e.g. 'playing football'), it can be helpful to explore with them why that is important to them. This helps avoid assumptions we can make based on our own views on the value of specific activities, and can also uncover broader values that could give inspiration for a host of other types of valued activities to consider. For example, playing football might be important to a young person because of the exercise (linked to a value around fitness), the social aspect (linked to a value around being part of a team and identifying as a group), stress relief (linked to a value around switching off or relaxing) or being outside (linked to a value about being in the elements). Depending on the underlying value, there will be different additional activities that fit with that value and are useful to consider when the original activity is not always possible.

Table 4.2. Distinguishing between values, valued activities and goals

	What are they?	Examples
Values	Ways you want to live your life, directions you want to go in, concepts that are important to you	Be respectful of others; nature; challenge myself

cont.

	What are they?	Examples
Valued activities	Specific behaviours that are important to you because they link to your values, and/or have an immediately identifiable sense of reward associated with them	Sketch; watch favourite TV show; play with younger sibling
Goals	A specific target that can be achieved	Walk the dog twice a week; join a drama club; redecorate my bedroom

However, we suggest that you don't get too worried about this if a young person finds it easier to identify activities than the values behind them. Our experience suggests it's not critical to distinguish, as long as the young person has understood the principle of Brief BA ('doing more of what matters' to them), is able to work out what does matter to them, and then starts making changes and doing activities that are in line with their values.

Troubleshooting

Many new Brief BA therapists tell us they worry about young people not being able to identify their personal values. In practice, we have found this is hardly ever the case. Remember, you will have been talking about 'what matters to you' (i.e. values) from the very start of Brief BA, so this language will not be wholly unfamiliar and you will have built up a good understanding of the young person by Session 3 as part of you getting to know them. All this means you will have laid the foundations for talking about values, and already have some ideas about what might be important for the young person. However, there are times when you can face challenges identifying values in Session 3, so we have given some suggestions for troubleshooting these in Table 4.3.

Table 4.3. Challenges with identifying values and how to troubleshoot these

The young person struggles to identify any of their own values	The young person only identifies values in one life area that they want to work on
Identifying the young person's values is key to the Brief BA approach, so if this takes a little longer than expected, that is fine	Discuss finding a balance of activities that relate to different life areas, and help young people make links between the things they are doing and their values
Young people might not be able to identify values immediately; it may require some thinking time – consider setting this as homework	Consider how a variety of activities can still be in accordance with the values they most want to work towards, but how some can also tap into other values (e.g. having a revision group with friends fits the 'education' value of doing well in exams, and the 'friends' value of spending time with them)
You may be able to make tentative suggestions based on activities they have rated highly on Achievement, Closeness, Enjoyment and Importance	Revisit the idea of a 'balance', and the need to get the 'feel-good' factor from different areas of life to make it more sustainable
You can use the worksheet examples to see if any of these fit for your young person	

Sometimes a value can feel particularly emotive, such as a young person who is not allowed contact with biological parents (for safeguarding reasons) wanting to feel closer to them. Being sensitive but realistic about feasible valued activities means you can often still find a way to help a young person towards this. In this example, the young person may identify that writing a letter to their mum, speaking with their foster parents about their biological family and looking at family photos might all be possible value-based activities. It is critical that the young person is always the driver of identifying values and valued activities, so these are rewarding for them.

CHAPTER 5

Brief BA Sessions 4 and Beyond

Doing More of What Matters

In this chapter, we will look at how to move to the most practical stage of Brief BA, where the focus is on the young person *planning* and then (most importantly) *doing* activities that relate to their own personal values. There is less new content here, but it's expected that you will be regularly referring back to the ideas we've covered in the earlier chapters of Part 2.

Moving from values to valued activities

- **Young person:** 'Brief BA helped me to work out what mattered to me and that by doing these things I could improve my mood.'

Once you have identified at least one or two values the young person feels are important to them, the next step is using these to plan how value-based activities can be incorporated into their everyday life. This is where you can be creative! Many values offer almost endless possible valued activities. For example, consider the different behaviours that might fit with 'being a good friend' and how this can vary depending on who the friend is, the kind of relationship the young person has with them, where they live, what is going on for them at the moment, the limits of what is possible for them to do right now, and their own personal views on what behaviours a good friend would show, and so on and so on! Brainstorming as many options that come to mind can help a young person see that even with the constraints of their current life (whether that's family rules, financial restrictions, academic requirements or health issues) they still have the ability to make some positive changes for themselves. Table 5.1 gives just some examples of how multiple activities could fit with a specific value.

Table 5.1. Linking values to valued activities

Value: Getting fit	Value: Doing well in school	Value: Getting along with mum and dad
Possible activities: Walk to college Join the boxing club at lunchtime Help out with youth club Join mum at her yoga class Give granddad a hand with his garden Download five-minute fitness exercises on my phone Meet Ramesh at the skate park	Possible activities: Do my homework the day it's set Ask Geography teacher to help me with assignment Get Maths revision guide Put my phone in other room when I'm studying Go to the library after school while I'm waiting for my lift	Possible activities: Go to the weekend family meet-up Use my headphones when listening to music Take my dirty plates down to the kitchen Go for a drive with dad

Breaking things down, starting small and aiming for success

Young person: 'It felt relaxed, not really pressured or anything. We went at my pace.'

The biggest problem most people (of any age) face when aiming to do things that matter to them is being too ambitious. For example, someone wanting to get fit will aim to go to the gym three times a week, or someone wanting to eat more healthily will aim for a complete detox diet. These aspirations are commendable, but by setting such big aims, the chance of failure increases.

Most activities people come up with can usually be broken down into smaller steps towards the bigger activity. For example, cooking a meal for the family might be a valued activity linked to a young person's passion for cookery and new cuisine. It might also link with a value around spending time with their family and being helpful to their parents. While the valued activity of cooking a meal for the family may be too ambitious, it can be broken down into a number of smaller activities:

- Telling the family about the plan
- Asking dad if he can help with the meal
- Choosing a recipe that is interesting but not too tricky, and one that everyone will eat
- Deciding on any side dishes or accompaniments
- Picking a night to cook
- Making a shopping list
- Going shopping for ingredients
- Letting everyone know when dinner is so they are home
- Doing homework the day before to free up the next evening
- Cooking the meal itself
- Agreeing who does the washing up!

Everybody falls into the trap of being too ambitious in their activity planning at some point, including ourselves, both in and out of the therapy room. But once you know this tendency, you can actively aim for the opposite – breaking activities down into their smallest components. This is especially important when working with depressed young people, who may be extremely sensitive to failure (or perceived failure), so avoid setting up tasks that are too difficult. As we will discuss further in Chapter 9, young people are still developing their cognitive skills for planning and evaluating tasks, so may need additional support to help identify sub-components and stages of a larger activity, and to organize these into a meaningful order. To help a young person understand how to start small, it is useful to say this from the outset, such as in the example below:

Therapist: 'The two most important things about valued activities are: number 1, that they are actually things you want to do (not just things you think you should do), and number 2, that they are achievable. We want to add in small changes to your life that you can keep building on, rather than aiming for something big that's hard to do or keep doing. The small changes are going to be much easier to keep doing, and over time they all add up to make a big difference in how much reward you're getting from life.'

Table 5.2 gives some examples of how larger activities can be broken down into smaller, but still value-based, activities.

Table 5.2. Linking values, valued activities and steps

Value	Larger activity	Smaller activity steps towards this
My health and wellbeing	Relaxation: meditate daily	• Find time in schedule to meditate • Look up brief meditations online • Download meditation app • Set reminder on phone • Find earphones to listen undisturbed • Turn phone to airplane mode
Politics	Join a protest march	• Look online at organizations to join • Sign up to mailing list • Find out date of local march • Check with mum • Ask cousin to go with me • Check train times
The environment	Reduce my use of plastic	• Research strategies to limit plastic use • Talk to family about this to share ideas • Watch documentary of someone's experience of trying to limit plastic use • Find sports water bottle in the garage • Sign petition for supermarket to limit plastic packaging

Valued activities in sessions

- **Young person:** 'It was nice to talk to my therapist about something I enjoy; I liked how they seemed to actually care what I'm into.'

When planning activities, remember the key motto, 'No activity is no activity', including your sessions! We are all engaging in an activity every minute of the day, whether we realize it or not (including ourselves as Brief BA therapists). Your time together in sessions is a fantastic opportunity to do valued activities, both to help the young person see the link between what they do and how they feel, and to scaffold the practice of this outside your sessions. The fact that you can do valued activities even within the constraints of your sessions will model to the young person that there is almost always a way to do more of what matters to them.

Remember, the fact that the young person has come back to your sessions suggests that the Brief BA work itself is a valued activity and they are likely to have some kind of value relating to getting better, helping themselves or feeling well. Highlight and provide reinforcement for this to the young person, as recognizing current activities as value-based can increase the level of reward associated with them.

We suggest that all Brief BA therapists should be working with their clients to plan and engage in valued activities in sessions, as well as outside them. Again, this is where you can be creative! There will understandably be limits on what is practical given your specific setting (e.g. time, location, resources available), but it is amazing how many valued activities are possible when you think outside the artificial constraint of talking rather than doing. Table 5.3 shows just a few examples of valued activities that have been completed in our Brief BA sessions.

Table 5.3. Valued activities in the therapy session

Value	Valued activity in session
Live music	Changing phone app to current location to find local live music events
	Texting a friend to see if they want to go to a music festival
	Checking out the dates that tickets are released
Rugby	Teaching Brief BA therapist the basic rules of Rugby League
	Showing Brief BA therapist how to throw a rugby ball
	Signing up for the local rugby team's mailing list on fixtures and events
Art	Drawing values rather than writing them
	Bringing in a sketch book to show Brief BA therapist their work
	Taking a 15-minute walk round the building with Brief BA therapist, looking at the artwork on the walls

Most young people will enjoy sharing their passions with an interested, curious audience; this can be you! It doesn't matter if you have no knowledge of the area; sometimes this can be a good thing as you are a willing learner. This gives the young person the opportunity to experience being in the expert role, which helps strengthen the teamwork ethos of Brief BA, and highlights the young person's strengths.

Top tip: Think about the things you've heard from young people that they are interested in, or spend a lot of time doing...how much do you really know about that topic? What could they teach you? Even if it's not something you're naturally interested in yourself, how might sharing their knowledge help you get to know the young person better, and what is rewarding for them?

When you engage in a young person's valued activities during a session, keep an eye out for changes in their affect (e.g. becoming more animated, talking more, looking and sounding brighter). If you see any of these changes, share this with the young person and ask them about their mood and remind them of the link between doing things that matter, and getting that 'feel-good factor' from life.

- **Therapist:** 'You know, when we were talking about [valued activity] just now I noticed you seemed more energetic, and you were smiling a bit and your voice got more animated. It looked as if talking about one of your favourite activities had an impact on your mood – how did that feel?'
- **Young person:** 'Yeah, I guess it's nice to talk to someone who's actually interested but doesn't know this all already... Mum doesn't have a clue and when I mention anything about [valued activity] her eyes just glaze over [small laugh].'
- **Therapist:** 'And how would you say your mood is now, compared to before we started talking about that?'
- **Young person:** 'Umm, a bit better probably? Not like amazing or anything, but it felt...good I guess.'
- **Therapist:** 'That's great to hear. You know how in Brief BA we say "No activity is no activity"? Well, that includes talking – it's an activity, too, so it looks as if talking about [valued activity] is probably a valued activity for you. Are there any other activities that fit with your values that we could try out together in our sessions?'

Clinician question: The room I use for my Brief BA sessions is pretty small and dull. How can I do valued activities in session?

Be creative, there is always a way! Sometimes you need to think outside the box – you might find problem-solving a helpful tool for this (see later in the manual). Think about how you can make use of the resources and environment even if this isn't your standard approach to a session. You might try some of the following:

- Bring some materials with you to the session to facilitate an activity (e.g. blank paper and pens for a young person to teach you how to write Japanese, or to explain a science experiment they are trying at school)
- Ask the young person to bring in something relating to their values that you can use in session (e.g. their sketch book, a story they've been working on, their favourite music)
- Make use of facilities nearby that fit for a valued activity (e.g. a badminton court, an art room, a library)
- Book a room big enough for them to show you their dance routine or Pilates exercises (you might need to bring some sportswear yourself!)
- Bring a laptop or use a room with a computer in it for internet access
- Look at photos and videos the young person wants to show you on their phone
- Take the topic of 'in session valued activities' to supervision to brainstorm ideas with others.

Valued activities outside sessions

Young person: 'I liked the timetable activities that I then followed throughout the day and felt achievement from every tick.'

Young person: 'I had a timetable that was like enjoyment, achievement and reflecting on my day, I could reflect on, actually things weren't that bad. I could also plan when I was gonna, for example, do a piece of homework and then have fun time. So it was almost, so it, it was balanced and it wasn't all play, it wasn't all work, so I was happier.'

Although doing activities in session is a great way of modelling that doing things differently can help people feel differently, it's essential that the young person also does this when they are not with you. This is key for the following reasons:

- Your sessions only make up a tiny fraction of their time (e.g. 1 hour out of 168 a week!)
- They need to develop the skill to plan and engage in valued activities without you.

Young people have different preferences for how they'd like to plan and timetable their valued activities. Some find the activity log useful, and will write in activities as a plan on this. Others prefer to use the life areas, values and activities (LAVA) worksheet and make a separate list of valued activities with specific details on when and where they could do these, then add them to their activity log when they've completed them. Some young people make use of other scheduling systems they already use, such as reminders on their phone, adding it to their school planner in the same way they do with their homework, or other kinds of diary or reminder systems. It really doesn't matter how these activities are planned; the key is that the method is a successful reminder and motivator while being flexible and acceptable.

If a young person is willing to involve others in helping them plan and engage in valued activities, this is where parents, carers and other important adults can be really useful. This works particularly well for activities that align with other people's values, as they tend to have a vested interest in helping the young person do these! As a Brief BA therapist, you can help important adults understand that a balance of activities (as well as those that fit with the adult's view of what the young person should be doing) is important for overall wellbeing.

Between-session work for the therapist and others

In the same way you expect the young person to undertake work between Brief BA sessions, you should also expect to do some between-session work. This is important to emphasize the collaborative nature of Brief BA, and to balance the need to have autonomy over looking after their mental health, with an appropriate level of support from the adults around them. Young people with more severe depression symptoms may require a greater degree of support from others at the beginning of therapy, which can be tailed off as their symptoms and functioning improve.

Between-session tasks for a Brief BA therapist may include activities such as:

- A phone call to parents to update and explain a homework task
- Contact with school or college to encourage support for the young person
- Exploring an app the young person uses to consider how it could be helpfully used in therapy
- Learning more about a young person's interest or hobby to consider ideas for valued activities around this
- Planning possible valued activities to complete in the next session.

Parents and carers may also have between-session tasks, such as:

- Meeting with school or college to discuss the best ways to support the young person
- Researching local clubs or resources to support a valued activity (e.g. finding out where the nearest rock climbing wall is)
- Making changes to the young person's bedroom to facilitate good sleep (e.g. buying new curtains)
- Taking the young person food shopping and discussing food choices
- Spending time with the young person doing a valued activity.

If a young person wants a parent or other important adult to do some work between sessions in order to help them make progress, it's important that this is checked out and agreed with the adult. Contracts may be a way of doing this that can be brought in earlier than Session 6 if needed (we talk more about contracts later on in the manual).

Troubleshooting

■ **Young person:** 'Sometimes it was hard to do things, even though I knew they would help… I just didn't have the energy.'

It's useful to remember that if it was simple to change behaviours when feeling depressed, the young person would have made these changes long ago and wouldn't need your help. Depression is a vicious cycle which is hard to escape from, so it can be challenging to attempt new activities, get enough support to be able to do these, and to sustain changes over a period of time. If you've tried using the Brief BA techniques yourself, you'll probably have noticed that it's remarkably easy to put off valued activities, run out of time for them, or forget them altogether. Now imagine if you were battling against the symptoms of depression, as well as being at a developmental stage where your brain and body are still developing, and you have limited autonomy and independence. That would make it much harder, wouldn't it?

Challenges are to be expected, which is why starting small, planning activities well, and troubleshooting ahead of time are so important. There may also be difficulties from external influences that aren't possible to predict that mean activities can't go ahead or don't go to plan. This is particularly true when activities rely on other people's involvement (e.g. if the young person's valued activity is to go to the cinema with friends, this is likely to only be valued if friends agree to join them). For activities that involve others or may be susceptible to other external factors (e.g. weather, train times, opening hours), these need extra planning and initial steps to check they are feasible.

❓ **Clinician question:** What if a young person wants to engage in an activity I feel is harmful?

This happens less than you would expect if you focus on the young person's values. If they do suggest an activity you do not want to encourage (e.g. drug taking), discuss the values behind the activity and brainstorm alternative activities that still fit with that value (e.g. value = spending time with friends, activity = go to the skatepark together). It's also helpful to consider how these activities might be contrary to other values they hold (e.g. 'looking after myself'). Any suggestion of harmful activities should be taken to supervision to discuss sharing information with parents or professionals.

When a young person engages in an activity, but doesn't enjoy it:

- This is a possibility, especially in the early stages of Brief BA. Normalize this experience; enjoyment might take a little longer to come back
- Explore how the young person approached the activity – were they fully engaged? For example, did they go out with friends, but spent the whole time on their phone not speaking? If so, encourage them to engage more fully with the activity, for example the next time they go out with friends, they could leave their phone in their pocket and join in the conversation
- Discuss how important the activity is – does it really fit with their values?
    - If not, identify another activity
    - If it does fit with their values, compare and reflect on the difference between how the young person was experiencing the activities before and how they experience them now
    - Did they used to enjoy it before they were depressed?

- Discuss how some activities might be important and value-based, but not enjoyable (e.g. going for regular blood tests to monitor a health condition, in line with staying healthy)
- Highlight times where things were difficult but the young person did not avoid the activity.

Clinician question: What if the young person identifies an activity their parents or carers don't agree with?

This could happen if a parent has different values to their child. Be clear with parents about the rationale for Brief BA (i.e. doing more of what matters to the young person, not other people), and discuss why this activity is important to their child. You could also:

- Negotiate – are there any compromises that can be reached?
- Use contracts or problem-solving within a session to help facilitate discussion and compromise.

Remember, your primary aim is to support the young person to implement their values, but they have to be feasible to increase their experience of rewards.

There may be some instances where there is a conflict between a young person's values and your own which could get in the way of Brief BA progress. For example, one young person might identify that hunting and shooting animals are valued activities for them, while you might be personally opposed to such sports. You should use supervision to think about any possibilities like this, so you can consider how you would approach this in the therapy room. Our advice is to consider whether by working towards that value the young person is likely to experience greater reward from life. Usually the answer is yes. Wherever possible, we suggest you encourage engagement in valued activities even when they do not fit your personal views, as long as they are not likely to harm the young person or others. This is something you should take to supervision to ensure you are able to fully support the young person. It is important to remember that the foundations of good therapy are in your therapeutic alliance with a young person, so you will need to take such issues to supervision to ensure you are able to maintain a curious, encouraging stance in sessions, and be positive about any activities that are valued and meaningful to the young person. With an open attitude and curious exploration, it is almost always possible to identify the broader values that such activities relate to that you, as a Brief BA therapist, can more easily encourage.

Reviewing progress

Young person: 'The graph was good as I could see how I was doing each week and how things were changing.'

As we've mentioned throughout this manual, it's important to track the young person's progress by using ROMs at every session. This is a reminder to review this and to consider patterns or changes that are apparent once you have more than three weeks of data.

We suggest that you plot scores in a visual form, either by hand or electronically. Your service may use software that creates such graphs for you automatically when you input the data, but creating your own graph is easy and doesn't take long. Young people tell us that they like to see the questionnaires turned into this visual depiction of how they are doing, and many have asked to have copies for themselves.

Their new scores should be plotted at every session and compared against the previous ones. You should be regularly discussing these with the young person and be curious about any changes or lack of progress.

Below is an example of one young person's ROMs that suggest something changed for the worse between Sessions 4 and 5. This shows how reviewing a young person's symptom and functioning scores (from both self and parent report) can lead to new and important learning.

THE BENEFIT OF REVIEWING ROMS

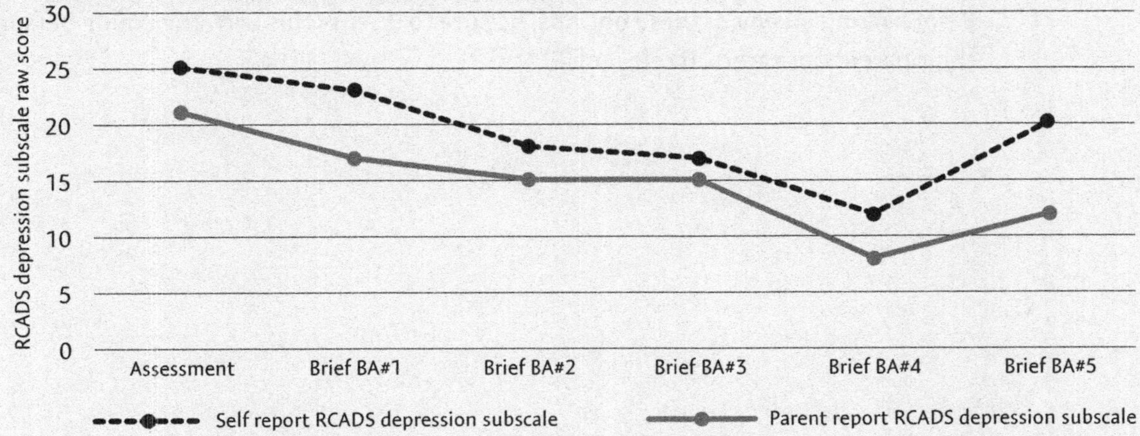

Figure 5.1. ROMs graph at Brief BA Session 5

Therapist: 'I can see that there has been a bit of a dip for you this week Nadia, with your scores for depression symptoms going up. Could we talk about what's been happening this week that might have led to this?'

Young person: 'Yeah... I had a horrible week at school... Keira and her mates decided to gang up on me and have basically been following me around and making my life hell. They threw my bag in the bin and ripped up my History homework, and keep saying horrible things about me to other people. It's been awful.'

Therapist: 'That really does sound awful, I'm sorry you've had to go through this. Have you spoken to anyone at school, or your parents about this?'

Young person: 'Not really...my friend Joelle knows it's been happening and said I should tell Miss Field, but I'm worried that might make it worse.'

Therapist: 'Well, thank you for telling me, I'm glad you felt able to and I'm sure we can find a way to make things feel better, not worse. Let's think together about what might be the best next step.'

? Clinician question: I feel really stuck with one of my Brief BA cases. What should I do?

- Use supervision to discuss your concerns. What makes you feel 'stuck'?

- Explore the ROMs for possible clues as to what might be stopping progress (e.g. sleep difficulties)
- Ask the young person for feedback: How are they finding the sessions? What do they think you could do differently that might help? It is okay to move session content forward. For example, if the young person identifies an issue that is getting in the way of changes they are trying to make, it would be useful to introduce problem-solving
- Discuss in supervision alternative treatment options; depending on your clinical context this might include inviting parents (or other adults) in to discuss ways they can help facilitate at home, a referral to another therapist who delivers an alternative evidence-based therapy, or to a child and adolescent psychiatrist to consider or review medication. Before acting on any of these options, be sure to discuss this with the young person (and their parents or carers, if relevant).

CHAPTER 6

Brief BA Session 6 (and Elsewhere When Needed)

Scaffolding and Support

Problem-solving

- **Young person:** 'I liked that I was able to find a logical solution and help for the problems I was facing.'

Problem-solving is a straightforward, intuitive way to approach a difficulty. Should be obvious, right? Well, think about a time when you've felt down, anxious, exhausted or struggling to concentrate. Chances are you've found it difficult to identify practical strategies that would help in that situation, because it's hard to think clearly when things are tough. Also, as we will discuss further in Chapter 9, some of the cognitive skills involved in problem-solving can be affected by depression as well as being skills most young people are still developing.

This means that having a practical and visual flow chart to use as a concrete problem-solving tool can really help. It also helps you, as a Brief BA therapist, to have a tool to draw on when you encounter difficulties in your session. It can be difficult to think clearly when you come across therapeutic challenges in the moment, so this gives both the therapist and young person a tool to draw on, in and outside sessions.

Including problem-solving as a standard tool within Brief BA helps both the young person and therapist raise any issues that might be getting in the way of progress. This could be something as simple as the timing of session appointments (e.g. if they always clash with the young person's favourite lessons at school, so they are missing out on a valued activity), to difficulties within their relationships, family or academic life.

Problem-solving follows a series of logical steps. The first step involves identifying and clarifying the problem. Next is the most creative step – the aim is to generate as many different solutions as possible. At this stage, the 'solutions' don't need to be practical – you and the young person can brainstorm and see how many different 'solutions' you can list. Once you are satisfied that you have exhausted all the options, the next step is to evaluate each 'solution' by weighing up the advantages and disadvantages, the pros and the cons. Once you have done this you should be able to select the best solution and figure out how to carry it out. The solution is tested and then the outcome is evaluated. If the problem has been solved, hurrah! If it hasn't been solved, you now have new information that can help you generate other options or re-evaluate the original options.

One example of problem-solving is shown in Table 6.1. This was useful when Ahmed was struggling to know how to approach the challenge of improving his Science grades at school.

Table 6.1. Example of problem-solving

Problem-solving step	Details
Step 1: Identify the problem	Failing Science
Step 2: Identify solutions	1. Hire an impersonator to do my Science exams for me 2. Get a tutor 3. Drop out of school and join a band 4. Ask Mrs Tatu for some extra help 5. Go visit my sister at uni for a Science bootcamp
Step 3: Pros and cons of each solution	1. I wouldn't need to bother with Science homework any more, but hiring someone would be expensive; I'm likely to get found out; they might not know the right answers anyway 2. Tutors are expensive and I would have to fit it in around other things 3. This isn't likely to work or be helpful long term! 4. It would be awkward to ask for extra help but I think she would probably say yes, and I could get help at school 5. I'd enjoy learning from my sister but I don't think I'd be allowed to visit during school term
Step 4: Select a solution	Option 4: Ask Mrs Tatu for extra help
Step 5: Plan the solution	Speak to Mrs Tatu at end of Science lesson on Tuesday (period 3), just before break
Step 6: Do it!	Did it!
Step 7: Review	Felt awkward waiting at the end of class, but Mrs Tatu was pleased I was asking for help. Gave me some revision worksheets and suggested some videos to watch; arranged to go over recent topics in tutor time on Friday morning

Contracting

- **Young person:** 'The contracts handout was useful, thinking about a certain activity and then thinking of who can help me with that and what I need to do to make sure they can help me with it...like, I wanted to do a few things while my girlfriend was over so I needed to, like, kind of plan out what I could do and who I would need to ask.'

Like problem-solving, contracts are a simple yet effective tool. Simply put, they are a way of agreeing specific help from specific people, with clear details of what is involved. Many people with depression find it hard to ask for help from others, and young people often tell us that they feel a burden to their parents and don't want to add to this. We also often hear from parents that they are desperate to help their child feel better, but struggle to know what to do. A contract offers a practical tool to facilitate this discussion, and to obtain an agreement over the actions. This can then be reviewed in Brief BA sessions, to consider how this went and to problem-solve (see above) any difficulties.

As a therapist, you may well have ideas (hypotheses) about certain ways parents or carers could be useful in supporting a young person's Brief BA treatment. However, you should always check these ideas out with a young person before bringing them up with parents in the room:

- **Therapist:** 'You mentioned last week that you didn't want to ask your dad to help you redecorate your bedroom but that it would be a really valued activity, and I wondered if that might be something we could discuss with him today?'
- **Young person:** 'Ummm... I guess, as long as we give him the option to say no. I don't want him to feel like he has to fork out for loads of stuff he can't afford...'
- **Therapist:** 'Okay, so it sounds as if you're worried about putting him under pressure, and also how much it might cost. Maybe we could speak to him about it and see if there's a way to make this work for everyone? Or would you prefer for us not to talk about it with him?'
- **Young person:** 'No, I think it's okay to bring it up, I've just been a bit scared to do it myself in case he says no...but he was saying on the way here how he wanted to help.'

Managing disagreement

Most (if not all!) young people will, at some point, disagree with their parents or carers about something. This is completely normal and part of the developmental transition towards the autonomy and independence of adult life. Most parents have had years of experience of negotiating differences between their child's views and their own, as well as setting rules and expectations for family life. Your brief intervention is not aimed at changing long-standing patterns of behaviour and strongly held familial or cultural views, so you need to be aware of what is and isn't going to be possible for the young person within their current home set-up.

However, disagreements between a young person and their parents or carers can sometimes be a barrier to progress in Brief BA, if they hinder the ability for the young person to engage in valued activities. This is where you, as a Brief BA therapist, have an important role in helping identify such barriers and considering how to help address these.

Top tip: Make sure you have understood the full picture of any disagreement between the young person and their parent or carer that is getting in the way of Brief BA progress. This means hearing both sides of the story, rather than relying solely on the young person's report. If their parent or carer isn't able to join sessions in person (or the young person doesn't want them to), suggest a phone call or email to talk through the issue before deciding on an action plan with the young person.

Sometimes the disagreement might be with other adults involved in the young person's life. This could be with school staff (there might be particular tensions between the young person and specific members of staff, while other school staff have a more positive relationship with them), or with youth workers, social care teams or other professionals involved in the young person's care.

The behavioural principles underlying Brief BA can be very helpful in managing disagreements. For example, even if a young person and parent do not agree about a specific valued activity, there might be examples in their discussion of this that are more aligned with each other. Positive reinforcement of these aspects can help them consider ways to build on this rather than focus on areas of tension. Modelling a calm, problem-solving approach to disagreements can also give a family an example of how to discuss differences of opinion without arguing or fighting. For some young people, parents and other adults, this may not be a common experience.

If a disagreement is getting in the way of the young person making progress in Brief BA, you will need to work on this. However, some disagreements are expected in life (we won't always get on well with everyone we meet), and there might be ways to work around some challenges. For example, if a young person doesn't find their tutor very supportive at school, there might be another school staff member who can give some extra guidance and check in regularly.

When to use these tools

Problem-solving and contracts are included in Session 6 because this is generally when parents or carers or other important adults are invited in. However, this doesn't mean you have to wait until Session 6 to use them! Think of these as tools in your Brief BA toolbox that you can draw on as needed.

Problem-solving might be helpful when:

- The young person is struggling to remember to complete their activity log
- There are some difficulties with engagement
- A friendship issue is getting in the way of them making progress
- A planned valued activity wasn't possible
- There is a difference of opinion in what they and their family want them to work on.

Contracts can be helpful whenever another person could facilitate a young person completing a valued activity. This includes you, as their Brief BA therapist, but remember that you won't be able to do this after their sessions end, so it's helpful for the young person to get used to asking others in their everyday lives for support of various kinds.

Top tip: If you're setting up a contract between the young person and someone else who is not in the room with you, make sure this is checked out with that person. Think about how it feels when someone volunteers you to do something without asking; even if you might be happy to help, it's much nicer to be asked! Think about how you can do this in the session (e.g. having the person in the room, the young person calling or messaging them), or set up a plan for the contract to be checked out with the other person afterwards. This could be you doing the checking, or (preferably) the young person themselves.

CHAPTER 7

Brief BA Sessions 7 and Beyond

Keeping Things Going

Reviewing progress and thinking ahead

As you progress through Brief BA sessions with a young person, you should start to see positive changes in how they are spending their time, and how they are thinking about their choice of activities. Recognize the success they have made, but also your own achievements at helping them get to this point.

You may be feeling pleased (and relieved) that you have managed to build a good relationship with the young person, and that they are coming back for future sessions. These are all things to be proud of, and you should share this progress in supervision. Many people feel they should only take problems to supervision, but you can learn a lot from discussing successes and what you did to enable them.

It's also possible that you may not be seeing the progress you'd hoped for by this stage, or the young person has hit a set-back. It can feel demoralizing and make it difficult to keep going. Supervision is essential when you're feeling like this, to help you manage your own emotions, but also to look at what is happening for that young person and how your Brief BA sessions could be adapted to be more useful. Sometimes it's also just about 'holding the hope' and being realistic about what progress looks like for each young person, and over what time frame this can be expected. For example, if you are working with a young person whose parent is terminally ill, you are unlikely to see the same improvements across Brief BA sessions compared to others whose circumstances are less challenging.

As you get to know the young person better, make sure you are linking back to things they've told you, and drawing on previous examples you can both learn from. It can be tempting to relax and perhaps reduce the effort you're putting into Brief BA sessions as you and the young person begin to feel more comfortable, but this is actually an opportunity for you both to maximize the gains that can be achieved in the remaining time you're working together.

- **Young person:** 'It felt like my therapist really listened...and remembered, so instead of forgetting and just saying "How are you today?", she'd ask about maybe a specific subject at school or a party that was coming up, and then she brought it up at the next session.'

As you become more comfortable with each other, you can use this trust to consider planning (and doing) valued activities that are a little more challenging for the young person. It's also a good time to revisit how others can help and support Brief BA, now that the young person is more familiar with you and what the work involves.

Building autonomy and independence

Young person: 'Brief BA gave me my own strategy to deal with low mood and gave me independence to do it.'

Brief BA is a relatively short intervention, focusing on building positive reinforcement for healthy, non-depressed behaviours into a young person's everyday life. This needs to continue after you finish working together, so you will need to build their ability to do this independently over the course of sessions. It's normal to feel like you are offering quite a lot of support, encouragement and suggestions at the start of Brief BA, which might be evident in the amount you are contributing to the session in relation to the young person's input. This should change as you get further into the treatment, so young people take a much more active role in later sessions. This often requires a deliberate 'sitting back' by the Brief BA therapist, as our desire to help can sometimes mean we offer lots of well-intentioned suggestions and support. While this might help in the short term, this does not help the young person build skills in helping themselves, which is needed for long-term, sustainable improvement.

Here are some strategies for building autonomy in Brief BA:

- Ask the young person for more input into sessions as they progress
- Listen to or watch back your session. Were there any opportunities to increase the young person's input, or to encourage their autonomy with taking Brief BA forward that you could have built on more? Bring these to the next session
- Give enough space for young people's suggestions or responses. Don't jump in too soon with your own
- Reflect back any instances of increasing independence with Brief BA work that you notice in a session
- Discuss in supervision how it feels to sit back and let a young person do more in a session.

Progress in Brief BA is by the very nature of the treatment, behavioural. This means that the young person themselves will have had to *do things differently* in order to *think and feel differently*. It's helpful to emphasize this, as it highlights that they have been responsible for the changes and progress, not you! It also gives them confidence that they will know how to keep making progress after your sessions finish.

Relapse prevention

Young person: 'I know I can keep going on my own now. Brief BA has given me strategies to cope.'

Towards the end of Brief BA, there should be an increasing focus on how to maintain any changes that have happened, or to problem-solve around why change hasn't been possible. Most of us work within time-limited settings where a specific number of sessions are agreed at the outset of therapy; with Brief BA this is suggested to be eight sessions plus a review around a month later. It is important to be clear with young people and their parents or carers as you come towards the end of your sessions with them, whether or not there is the possibility of further sessions or of seeing you again in the future. Most of the time you won't be able to see the young person much longer than originally planned, and this can actually be a good thing (see 'Endings in therapy' in Chapter 8).

Top tip: It is helpful to name the session number and how many sessions are left, each time you meet the young person. This is especially useful if you are in an environment where you may see the young person in more informal ways. Make sure you are distinguishing between the Brief BA treatment sessions and the review. It might be helpful to say something like the example below.

- **Therapist:** 'It's good to see you again. This is our sixth Brief BA session, so after today we will have two more sessions, then a final review session about a month after that to see how things are going. We still might see each other around school after that, but we won't be meeting one-to-one like this for Brief BA work.'

If there is already a plan for what will happen after your Brief BA sessions end, make sure you remind the young person of this. Similarly, if there is something else that will define the last time you meet (e.g. if the young person is moving away to study elsewhere, or your role will be finishing in that team), also remind them of that end point and how many more times you'll meet before this.

At the same time as reminding them of the number of Brief BA sessions left, you should also be working with the young person to plan how they can keep things going after you finish. This is really about distilling the key ideas of Brief BA and making sure they have a plan of how to continue using them in future.

Some simple techniques can help, including:

- Completing a 'Healthy Me' worksheet in session
- Creating their own bespoke one-page summary of Brief BA (e.g. spider diagram, thought bubbles etc.)
- Keeping copies of Brief BA worksheets in a dedicated folder
- Taking photos of key Brief BA ideas or worksheets and saving these on their computer or phone
- Checking the parent's or carer's understanding of the Brief BA techniques covered, and asking them for ideas of how to keep things going
- Planning in regular time to check in and review progress, ideally with someone else (e.g. family member, teacher, youth worker).

Remember, although Brief BA sessions are time-limited, by helping the young person develop new strategies to 'do more of what matters' you are supporting long-term change.

CHAPTER 8

Ending Therapy and Living a Valued Life

- **Young person:** 'I'm worried what will happen when Brief BA stops, in case I go back to how I was before.'

Where are we now?

Our aim in Brief BA is to help the young person re-engage with the rewards in their life, to increase valued activities and positive reinforcement, and improve their symptoms and day-to-day functioning. Brief BA is designed to be a time-limited and focused intervention, and so it is important to be clear about what will happen when your time-limited intervention comes to an end. The most desirable outcome is that the young person has made sufficient improvement, and has re-engaged with and is managing their usual activities (education or work, friendships, family life).

In our practice, we routinely offer a follow-up session one month after the final session of Brief BA. This allows us to check in on the young person and to find out how they are doing. If all is well, the optimal outcome is to discharge them completely. However, this is not always possible, even if they have made progress in Brief BA.

Handing over or referring on

Sometimes a brief intervention will not be sufficient to help a young person recover from depression, and further help is needed. Brief BA will not be effective for all young people, and the options for what happens next are likely to depend on your specific service. If the young person has engaged in Brief BA but is still feeling depressed, it's important to find the right route for further help. This should be part of overall care planning for this young person and discussed in supervision and with your team to consider best options. These should also be discussed with the young person and their parent or carer in the review session.

During treatment new problems can emerge or old problems may re-emerge. For example, once the dominant symptoms of depression have reduced, young people sometimes report that this has awoken dormant symptoms of anxiety – now that their depression is not keeping them in their room or at home, they are fearful or worried. Their fears are not new, but they were not present when the young person was at home avoiding life. This may need to be the focus of future work after Brief BA is completed.

If someone else is taking over to deliver further treatment, wherever possible there should be a joint meeting between the young person (and parent or carer, if appropriate), the Brief BA therapist and the new clinician. It's helpful to outline the work completed in Brief BA (including sharing any information the young person feels happy with), along with what the young person has found helpful and what further input they feel would be useful.

Endings in therapy

As a likely source of stable positive reinforcement, the Brief BA therapist should expect that the end of therapy might be challenging for a young person as this source of reinforcement will be lost. To help young people understand the brief nature of the work and to encourage them to aim for independent progress after the sessions end, the therapist should agree the number of sessions at their first appointment, and review this regularly throughout (e.g. 'Today is session x of xx, so we'll have xx more treatment sessions after today'). It is also important to make this clear to all involved in the care of the young person, so there are realistic expectations.

It can be helpful to consider these points:

- Clarify the tailing-off nature of the final sessions. Have bigger gaps between appointments towards the end, to help the young person try out making progress independently
- Emphasize the expectation that progress will continue after the sessions end, as new strategies take time to become familiar and impact on mood and functioning
- Explicitly discuss who can help support the young person's progress once the sessions end, and how this will be put in place (e.g. regular catch-up with mum to check in, meeting with tutor once a week etc.)
- Be mindful that young people who lack supportive adults in their life and/or who have experienced loss of important sources of positive reinforcement previously may find the ending of therapy particularly hard. Bring such cases to supervision.

Replacing therapist reinforcement

Young person: 'I miss being able to talk about my week to someone who really cared.'

As you've heard throughout this manual, the Brief BA therapist is a key reinforcer for healthy behaviour. If this has worked well, it's likely that the young person will find your sessions a positive, rewarding experience, and therefore ending these sessions could be a potential loss of reward.

To address this, it's important that you look for sources of this reinforcement from the young person's everyday life and support network, so they do not experience a loss of reward at the end of therapy.

Key sources of reinforcement that are sustainable after the end of Brief BA include:

- Creating a structure of regular planned activities that are known to be rewarding
- The young person encouraging and praising themselves for their continued efforts, recognizing their progress
- Parents or carers who can continue to encourage the young person to engage in valued activities and provide positive reinforcement.

Some young people (and their parents or carers) worry about how they will manage without the Brief BA therapist input. However, the fact that Brief BA is so focused on changes in the young person's day-to-day activities means that any positive changes in mood can be directly attributed to these behavioural changes. These, necessarily, have been done by the young person, so the Brief BA therapist can reflect this to emphasize that this is possible after Brief BA sessions end.

Service specifics

Every service setting will have different procedures around the end of therapy (e.g. a maximum number of sessions, other kinds of support available in the same team, referral routes and options for other services), so you will need to know what these are before you are asked by the young person or their parent! These can change over time, so it's a good idea to keep up to date with this information, and also ensure you have the correct contact details for other services in the area that the young person could access. Often there is some kind of end of treatment care planning review that services require; this can easily be built into the Brief BA review session.

Clinician question: How do I manage the ending of Brief BA sessions?

- Be clear about the number of sessions from the start, and refer to this through your work (e.g. 'Today is session 4 of 8')
- Be aware that you may be a source of positive reinforcement for the young person, and that ending sessions may remove this. It is important to find other ways to get this reinforcement from their environment
- Some people may find endings harder than others. Young people who have experienced interpersonal losses, and those who have established a strong therapeutic relationship with you, may find this more difficult
- Parents often worry about sessions ending. Be clear about how they can get support after your sessions end, and signpost to the resources in the worksheets
- Be realistic. Use the 'Healthy Me' worksheet to discuss potential set-backs and how they can use their new skills to overcome these
- Reinforce that the changes that have been made are down to them (to give them the confidence that they can continue to do this after sessions have finished).

Reviewing and using ROMs can help manage endings, as shown in this example.

Therapist: 'So I remember at Session 8 we talked about how you and your dad were worried about how to keep things going once our sessions ended, and this was shown in your symptom scores going up a bit. It looks like today's scores are pretty low; what's changed since we last met?'

Young person: 'Back then I didn't think I could do it on my own, but that's pretty much what I've done over the last month so I feel more confident about it now.'

Therapist: 'That's great to hear! Can you talk me through what you've been doing that's helped you feel more confident?'

- **Young person:** 'I've been making sure I have a balance of fun and relaxing stuff each day, even when I've got a lot of college work on, and planning in when I can do bigger stuff like going out with my friends. I've not let myself put things off so much, especially if I know I'll feel better getting them done or helping others out. And generally I've been thinking more about doing things I actually care about rather than stuff that's not as important.'

- **Therapist:** 'Sounds like Brief BA in action, well done! Like you say, you've been doing this over the last month without us meeting, so it shows you carry the Brief BA work on even though our sessions are ending.'

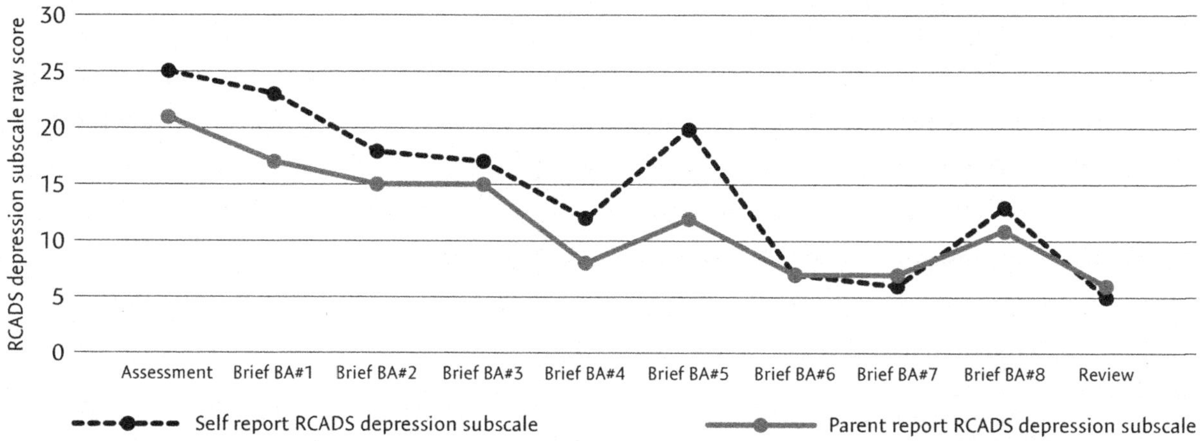

Figure 8.1. ROMs graph at end of Brief BA

You will need to think about how to say goodbye at the end of your work together. Everyone has different ways of doing this, and you should ask the young person before the final meeting how they might like to mark this end. Before this, be clear what is and isn't okay to do in your specific setting, as well as with your own personal boundaries. In some settings a goodbye hug can be appropriate, but it might not be in others (and even if it is, you might not want to do this). Also make sure you know your service policy on whether you can accept any thank you gifts (and talk in supervision about whether you'd feel okay accepting one, even if you're allowed), in case the young person brings one for you.

Young people and their parents or carers can find it hard to say goodbye, but it might also be difficult for you. This is a natural response to building a good working relationship with a young person and enjoying working together, but it can also feel hard to end if a young person is still struggling with depression symptoms and you aren't able to do any more. This can lead to you feeling as if you have failed as a therapist and make it hard for you to maintain optimism in your final sessions. Talk about your upcoming endings in supervision to make sure you have the time, space and support to explore these feelings without it affecting your clinical work.

All of these things will help you feel more prepared for the ending, and better able to support the young person in this.

Ways a young person may want to say goodbye can include:

- Writing a goodbye letter or card
- Shaking hands

- A hug
- Saying 'goodbye'
- Walking out without looking back.

It can be helpful to send a closing letter to the young person and/or parents and carers outlining the work you've completed and what will happen next. This will give you a chance to personally thank them for the work they put into sessions, clarify that Brief BA has now finished, and confirm who they should contact in the future.

Clinician question: Can I offer any top-up sessions after the review?

> This depends on your setting, and what the rationale is for this. Many services work on the basis of closing and discharging young people at the end of therapy, so you may not be able to see them again unless they are re-referred.

If you are able to offer them, Brief BA top-up sessions could be used if the young person starts to feel depressed again or has a particular set-back, and it feels like a discrete number of sessions (usually one or two) would help them get back on track. These sessions could revisit concepts you covered in the original Brief BA sessions, to help them make use of the techniques you covered.

A Brief BA top-up session might involve:

- Re-capping the rationale for Brief BA
- Problem-solving anything that has prevented maintenance of their progress
- Revisiting their personal values and whether there have been any changes that could give them ideas about valued activities moving forwards
- Referring to relapse prevention information (using the 'Healthy Me' worksheet)
- Considering who could help support them in continuing Brief BA without your input.

PART 3

THE THEORY AND RESEARCH BEHIND BRIEF BA (THE 'WHY')

This part of the manual is for those of you who are curious about Brief BA and want to take a closer look at the theories and research that are the building blocks of the treatment. If you are on a training programme and have to write a case report or essay about Behavioural Activation or depression in adolescents, the references and information here might be useful. We also thought that supervisors who come to Brief BA and who are experienced in other models of psychological therapy might like to find out a bit more behind the rationale for the Brief BA approach to treating depression.

To start, Chapter 9 provides a general introduction to the topic of adolescent depression and the challenges of identifying and treating depression in young people. It then illustrates how key features of Brief BA are designed specifically to meet these challenges.

Next, Chapter 10 highlights the essential task of getting to know the young person and keeping them safe. It focuses on engaging young people in psychological treatment and on collaboration with them and their parents or carers. It explains the concept of the therapeutic alliance or therapeutic relationship. In this chapter, we also discuss the evidence and science around the therapeutic alliance and on monitoring and managing risk. We explain why we use Routine Outcome Measures (ROMs) in Brief BA, and how this contributes to the quality of treatment and the safety of the young people who are in treatment.

In Chapter 11, we discuss the behavioural theory of depression. We explain how depression is maintained by avoidance and lack of positive reinforcement. We also describe how the behavioural theory of depression is used in Brief BA to help young people overcome their depression symptoms and increase positive reinforcement and rewards.

Chapter 12 focuses on the key role of values (i.e. 'what matters to you') in Brief BA. Helping young people identify what matters to them helps engagement and collaboration. Importantly it also allows the young person and therapist to identify valued activities, and structure activities linked to these to reduce avoidance and experience more rewards and positive reinforcement.

Chapter 13 highlights key therapeutic strategies that we use in Brief BA. These have been developed in a range of different psychological therapies and are used to treat a range of difficulties. Here we highlight the role of psychoeducation, goal setting, activity and mood monitoring, healthy habits, contracting and problem-solving.

Finally, in Chapter 14, we discuss and weigh up the evidence that supports the use of Brief BA for adolescent depression. This is really important because depressed young people deserve to be offered a safe and effective treatment. You may also be asked about the evidence for Brief BA when discussing treatment options with young people and families.

CHAPTER 9

The Unique Challenge of Adolescent Depression

Understanding depression

Depression is a mental health problem that is experienced by many people of all ages. However, the period of life when you are most likely to develop depression is in adolescence. At any time, between two and three per cent of adolescents are experiencing an episode of depression, and this figure is pretty much the same around the world (Polanczyk *et al.* 2015). As discussed earlier, depression that meets the criteria for a diagnosis (e.g. Major Depressive Disorder [MDD] or Persistent Depressive Disorder [PDD], also known as dysthymia) is much more than simply feeling sad. In fact, many young people with a depressive disorder do not say that they feel sad or unhappy.

There are three core symptoms of depression in adolescents:

- Sadness or low mood
- Irritability
- Anhedonia.

You already know what sadness and irritability mean. As outlined in Part 2, it is important to ask about both when you assess a young person with depression. Young people who do not feel tearful or sad often know that they feel angry and irritable with other people. Parents and teachers and friends may notice them being irritable but not know that this is a symptom of depression. Although many young people who do not have depression feel irritable some of the time, if this continues for more than two weeks and interferes with how they are able to manage their day-to-day life, it may be worthwhile considering if they have depression. Sometimes depressed young people stay away from other people because they get so quickly and easily annoyed. They worry that they will not be able to control their irritability and will end up upsetting other people.

'Anhedonia' is a symptom that most of us don't immediately recognize and might not realize is linked with depression. As we saw in Part 2, anhedonia means lacking enjoyment or pleasure. In our research (Watson *et al.* 2019) young people described anhedonia as feeling 'nothing at all', and their experience as 'flat' or 'empty' and their lives as 'grey'. Anhedonia has been described as a problem that is associated with a lack or deficit of rewards (e.g. Rømer Thomsen 2015). Closely linked to anhedonia, young people also report that they feel unmotivated, lack energy and feel separate from other people, and sometimes they feel isolated and alone (Watson *et al.* 2019). Anhedonia is of particular interest to us because around two-thirds of depressed young people report this

(Goodyer *et al.* 2017), and there is evidence that adolescents who have this symptom are less likely to benefit from psychological therapies (McMakin *et al.* 2012). Brief BA treatment directly targets the experience of anhedonia by aiming to increase pleasure and enjoyment (and thus rewards) through valued activities.

Other symptoms of depression are also distressing and disabling for young people. In a large study of 465 depressed young people, Goodyer *et al.* (2017) reported the frequency with which different symptoms were reported (shown in Table 9.1). More than 90 per cent of young people with depression reported problems with sleep, making this the most common symptom overall. Sleep problems include insomnia, that is, not being able to get to sleep, or waking early, or in the middle of the night and not being able to get back to sleep, and hypersomnia, that is, sleeping for too long. Some depressed young people also report that their sleep patterns are disturbed so they sleep during the day and are awake at night.

Table 9.1. Frequency of symptoms reported by young people with depression

Symptom	Frequency (%)
Sleep disturbance	92
Low or depressed mood	84
Disturbed concentration, indecision	75
Fatigue, lack of energy	73
Negative self-perceptions, excessive guilt	68
Anhedonia	65
Irritability	63
Appetite problems	61
Suicidal thoughts	60
Psychomotor problems (agitation or retardation)	55

Note: N = 465; symptoms *in italics* are core symptoms of MDD (DSM-5).

Source: Data from Goodyer et al. (2017)

The key challenges of adolescent depression

Challenge 1: There are not nearly enough trained clinicians who can offer conventional evidence-based psychological therapies. This means that there is a shortage of therapists and long waiting lists for treatment. Because of this, depression goes untreated for long periods of time, it becomes more severe, and young people miss more opportunities in their everyday lives.

Challenge 2: Only about half of young people who are offered other evidence-based treatment get better. This is very concerning. We used to think that recovery rates were higher, but recent reviews of the research evidence (e.g. Weisz *et al.* 2017) point out that more recent and better-designed studies show that psychological therapies for depression have more limited effectiveness.

Challenge 3: Many young people drop out of existing evidence-based therapies. For example, in a recent treatment trial of 465 depressed young people (Goodyer *et al.* 2017), 37 per cent dropped out of treatment before the end. We don't know why young people drop out of treatment, and it's likely to be for many different reasons.

What makes treating depression in young people so challenging?

Although depression is broadly similar in adults and adolescents, there are important things that make depression in young people challenging to treat. Many therapists assume that because adolescents are on their way to becoming adults, treatments designed for adults can be used with no specific changes. We think this is unhelpful and is often part of the reason why young people drop out of therapy. Understanding important aspects of depression in adolescents can help us design and then offer therapy in a way that is useful to young people.

There are some key issues to keep in mind when you start treatment with a depressed young person.

Young people are still developing

Although this is an obvious point, clinicians and therapists who work with depressed young people often overlook it. Adolescence is a time of life when we change and develop in many different and sometimes hidden ways. While it is easy to see the physical changes that happen, the psychological and emotional changes can be more difficult to observe. Over the past 20 years, our scientific understanding of how the adolescent brain develops has been hugely improved, and this new understanding provides essential background information for therapists working with young people.

FURTHER READING ON ADOLESCENTS AND THE DEVELOPING BRAIN

Blakemore, S. J. (2017) *Inventing Ourselves: The Secret Life of the Teenage Brain*. New York: Doubleday.

Maddox, L. (2018) *Blueprint: How Our Childhood Makes Us Who We Are*. London: Robinson.

Cognitive development

The development of the brain and cognitive abilities drives changes in how adolescents and adults understand themselves and other people. Different parts of the brain develop at different rates. During adolescence and early adulthood a key area of the brain that develops rapidly is the pre-frontal cortex. This area of the brain, which sits behind the forehead, is responsible for advanced thinking skills – including planning, organizing, controlling emotions and impulses, and making sense of experiences and deciding how to respond. These skills are collectively known as 'executive skills' in reference to their central and coordinating role (Blakemore and Choudhury 2006). Therefore, across adolescence young people's executive functioning develops and they become more skilful at these advanced thinking skills. They become better decision-makers, can more often inhibit their initial impulses, and are more easily able to anticipate future events and plan for these. They also develop more control over their thoughts, and this helps manage their moods and emotions.

Response to rewards

Adolescents also differ from adults in how they respond to rewards. Rewards elicit and provoke positive emotions, including joy, satisfaction, pleasure, excitement, enthusiasm and fulfilment, often immediately and intensively.

Rewards come in a range of different ways:

- Physical, e.g. food, drink, physical exercise
- Social, e.g. spending time with friends, praise, attention
- Indirect and symbolic, e.g. money
- Sensory, e.g. pleasing textures, sexual activity, music.

Typically, rewards capture adolescents' attention and are attractive and engaging. This can be inferred from their behaviours, for example increased interest, repeating the behaviour or seeking out and working for the reward. Heightened sensitivity to rewards encourages adolescents to explore their environment and seek out new experiences. This exploration and experience helps them learn and is integral to making the transition from childhood dependence to adult independence. However, enhanced sensitivity to reward can also increase adolescents' exposure to risk and danger (e.g. drugs, alcohol, risky physical activities), which, when linked with immature impulse control and executive functioning, also increases their vulnerability.

Response to rewards is also demonstrated on a neural level and changes over the course of adolescence (Forbes *et al.* 2010), and young people show greater neural activation than adults when they receive or anticipate a reward (Braams *et al.* 2015). When promised or given a reward (e.g. a chocolate drink), the brain becomes activated, and this is more pronounced in young people than in adults. However, there is evidence that young people with symptoms of depression have blunted responses to rewards compared to adolescents who are not depressed (Rzepa, Fisk and McCabe 2017). This means that their brains do not respond as strongly to rewards as those of young people who are not depressed. This neural blunting is consistent with adolescents' experiences of anhedonia, where they describe that their usual feelings of enjoyment and pleasure are absent or less intense. It is not known if problems experiencing rewards are a response to becoming depressed, or if this reward deficit exists before the onset of depression and increases the risk of depression. However, some theorists (e.g. Pizzagalli 2014) suggest that people who have an impaired or disrupted reward system are at increased risk of developing depression, and that an important cause of depression is impaired reward functioning.

Sensitivity to social cues

Young people are also highly sensitive and attentive to social cues. As they develop, they become better able to imagine what other people are thinking or feeling. This skill, known as 'mentalizing', allows adolescents to more accurately take or understand another person's perspective (Choudhury, Blakemore and Charman 2006). The social environment also changes how young people behave. Fascinating evidence from mock driving experiments shows that when they are interacting with other young people (or via a computer they believe that they are), they make more impulsive decisions and take more risks (Blakemore and Robbins 2012). Our own research shows that adolescents are highly attuned to their relationships with others. For example, Orchard, Pass and Reynolds (2019) found that although depressed young people typically describe themselves in highly negative ways ('I am worthless', 'I am useless', 'I am pathetic'), they manage to hold some positive attributes, all of which relate to how they get on with other people ('I am friendly', 'I am trustworthy', 'I am kind').

Adolescent development and depression

All these changes makes many new and exciting things possible. Young people discover their talents and interests, often begin romantic relationships, identify their ambitions and start to plan for a future, adult life. However, adolescents still have brains that are highly malleable. Depression interferes with young people's cognitive and emotional development in very direct ways, and we will discuss this at greater length below. Depression interferes with how young people describe themselves, the world around them and their futures (Beck 1979). It affects decision-making and can therefore essentially shape the future that the young person will have and the future self that they become. Depressed young people often feel hopeless, worthless, useless and unlovable. In this state of mind they are not in a good place to make important life-long decisions or answer important questions. This is why we need to make sure that therapy for adolescents who have depression takes account of their ongoing development and gives them opportunities to develop and grow into the people they want to become.

Brief BA has been designed specifically to adapt to the developmental changes across adolescence. We encourage young people to identify values that are their own as distinct from those of their peers and friends, parents and family, school and wider cultural context. We keep therapy simple but accept fully that this is not easy. Our worksheets are highly structured to help scaffold and support developing cognitive abilities.

Young people have less autonomy than adults

For legal and financial reasons young people have to rely on their parents or other carers for practical and emotional support. There are restrictions on what they do with their time, where they go and who they spend their time with. There are legal limits to the autonomy that any young person can have, and there are also individual family and cultural limits to a young person's freedom and autonomy. These can be a cause of friction within families and cultures.

Young people usually have to manage many different social, academic and family demands, which further limits their autonomy and freedom. As described above, during adolescence, friendships and relationships become extremely important. Young people become excruciatingly aware of how other people judge them. They become more self-conscious and hyper-aware of how they 'look' to others (Somerville 2013; Somerville *et al.* 2013). They compare clothes, hair, friendships, behaviours and interactions with others in real life and on social media. They monitor their surroundings for clues that they are acceptable and 'liked' by other young people. This process of social comparison is at its most extreme during adolescence, feeds engagement in online social media and 'real-life' social activities, and is often a source of emotional highs and lows.

School exams (usually at around the ages of 16 and 18) can become a huge and over-bearing fact of life. Teachers, parents and students feel under increasing and extreme pressure, and exams often begin to dominate their lives. As one young person said, 'Forget everything else, exams are your life' (quoted in Watson *et al.* 2019). Alongside academic pressures, many young people have part-time jobs, play competitive sport and are learning other skills, such as driving or a musical instrument.

In Brief BA, we recognize that the young person's autonomy is limited but that it is developing. Whenever possible, we engage parents and carers to make sure that they are able to support the young person emotionally and practically. We also review the balance of activities that young people are already doing, and work to increase the proportion of valued activities so that they achieve a more rewarding and sustainable balance.

Services for young people can be confusing and hard to access

Because it can be hard to recognize the signs of depression, it often takes months or even years before a young person, or their parent or carer, notices that they have a problem and thinks about asking for help. Then it is often not obvious who to go to for help. Although awareness of mental health problems is much greater now than it was 20 years ago, this has resulted in many different types of information and help being available, and varies from town to town and city to city. It is often not clear where to start asking for help. Most of the young people we see have had depression for around two years before they arrive at the clinic. Usually a parent has initially taken them to see their family doctor. Sometimes (but not often), they have already had some therapy or counselling. Sometimes, although anti-depressant medication alone is not recommended as the first line of treatment for young people with depression (NICE 2019), family doctors will have prescribed medication because they cannot find any more accessible treatment. Whatever treatment they have had or not had, by the time they get into our clinic young people who come for treatment for depression are still not feeling better.

Many problems accessing treatment for depression are created and maintained by a scarcity of formally trained psychological therapists. Brief BA is designed to be delivered by professionals who are not highly qualified and experienced psychological therapists. This means that many more people can learn to deliver Brief BA safely and well. Individuals who work in schools and primary care can learn the skills necessary to provide this brief treatment for adolescent depression under the appropriate supervision. The core ideas of Brief BA are simple and are supported by practical worksheets for each session. However, as discussed throughout this manual, although Brief BA is simple to understand, it is often not easy to deliver (as a therapist) or to use (as a young person). To deliver Brief BA safely and well it is important to understand the key principles of the treatment, to be able to engage a young person in treatment, and to be receiving (and using) regular clinical supervision.

The symptoms of depression directly interfere with treatment

Once young people with depression get offered therapy it can be very hard to start. Young people often find it difficult to get to the clinic, are uncomfortable and embarrassed to sit in a room with an adult who is a stranger, feel tongue-tied and unable to talk, and find it impossible to believe that things can change for the better. Ironically, the symptoms of depression (e.g. hopelessness, low motivation and cognitive problems) directly interfere with therapy and with recovery.

Poor sleep is the most common symptom that depressed young people report (see Table 9.1; Goodyer *et al.* 2017). Poor sleep is bad enough, but it has further negative consequences – fatigue, low energy levels, irritability, problems thinking and reduced motivation. Motivational problems make it hard to engage in treatment, to turn up to sessions, to carry out therapy tasks and to change. Thinking problems (also a symptom of depression) interfere with young people's ability to make decisions and make it especially hard for them to plan and take actions. After they leave a session, their memory and concentration problems often mean that they find it hard to remember what happened in the therapy session. This is why it is essential that therapists make it as easy as possible for young people to engage in and benefit from therapy.

Young people with depression also have a very specific problem with their *working memory* (see the box below for further reading on this). Working memory is a core cognitive system that is used to hold and manipulate information for a short period of time. For example, we use working memory when we need to hold a sequence of numbers in mind long enough to write them down, use them (e.g. make a telephone call) or enter them into a computer. Working memory is used to remember the specific numbers, and their order. Once the numbers are recorded or have been used, they no longer need to be held in working memory and can be discarded (forgotten), or transferred into another part of memory. Other day-to-day uses of working memory are remembering tasks ('What did I run upstairs for?'), shopping lists ('Was it bread or butter we've run out of?'), and following directions ('Did she say right at the traffic lights or straight on?').

Working memory develops during childhood and adolescence. It plays a crucial role in education and academic performance. It is particularly crucial when learning mathematics (e.g. doing mental arithmetic), learning to read and learning foreign languages. Problems with working memory make it hard to follow verbal instructions and interfere with tasks that require sustained attention and recall of previous steps. In fact, working memory strength in childhood is a better predictor of young people's academic performance than IQ (St Clair-Thompson and Gathercole 2006).

Recent evidence has demonstrated that compared to their non-depressed peers, young people with elevated symptoms of depression have impaired working memory (Fisk, Ellis and Reynolds 2019). We don't know if working memory is damaged temporarily during the period of depression and then recovers once depression has lifted, or if young people with poor working memory are more likely to become depressed. Either way, the problems that depressed young people have with working memory interfere with their schoolwork (which is often a cause of great distress), and are also a key obstacle in therapy. Working memory problems make it hard for young people to pay attention to their therapist, to hold information in mind and to transfer information into long-term memory so that it can be used to help recovery.

In Brief BA, we have designed worksheets for each session (see Part 4). These help to minimize demands on working memory. The central information that young people need is brief, simple and written down so it need not be held in mind. Key points are illustrated with pictures, diagrams and examples. There is space for young people to write down things that are important to them. There are also parallel parent worksheets so that parents can give practical support to the young person between sessions.

FURTHER READING ON WORKING MEMORY

Baddeley, A. and Hitch, C (1994) 'Developments in the concept of working memory.' *Neuropsychology* 8(4), 485. [The most influential account of working memory.]

Fisk, J., Ellis, J.A. and Reynolds, S.A. (2019) 'A test of the CaR-FA-X mechanisms and depression in adolescents.' *Memory 27*(4), 455–464. [This article shows that working memory is impaired in young people with symptoms of depression.]

Gathercole, S.E. and Alloway, T.P. (2008). *Working Memory and Learning: A Practical Guide for Teachers*. London: Sage. [Clearly describes the role of working memory in education.]

How does Brief BA help overcome the challenge of adolescent depression?

Our aim is to work with what depressed young people can do, rather than what they cannot do. We adapted Brief BA and developed this manual to help therapists who work with depressed young people to overcome the many obstacles and challenges outlined above. Brief BA is based on good evidence and uses simple and well-founded psychological principles. We have drawn on our clinical experience as well as our own research findings and well-established research by other people. We have also talked at length to young people about what it is like to be depressed and what helps their recovery. Parents and carers of young people have also told us about how adolescent depression affects them – we know that most parents and carers want to do whatever they can to help and support their child. Finally, but also very importantly, we have trained many individual therapists who work with young people and asked them what helps them to deliver treatment well, what they find difficult, and what they feel will help them do a good job and keep young people safe and able to overcome the problems that depression presents to them.

We know that working with depressed people is hard and can be discouraging. Our aim is to offer a brief, practical and effective therapy that therapists can learn quickly and then, with appropriate supervision, deliver compassionately and skilfully. Throughout this treatment manual we hope that therapists and their supervisors will find practical advice, support and encouragement.

Brief BA treatment is structured and time-limited. We hope that this is helpful to therapists and young people. Every part of the treatment is visible and explicit. In this section, each session or group of sessions that are part of the Brief BA treatment is discussed and we explain why they are designed that way. We hope that this will help you feel confident when you and a young person use Brief BA. If you want to find out more, please follow up the references mentioned below.

Table 9.2. Challenges of adolescent depression and how Brief BA approaches them

Key challenge of adolescent depression	Relevant Brief BA component
Ongoing development	Identifying values links with identity formation – who am I? Brief BA is simple, but not easy Include case examples of other young people
Limited autonomy	Work on a balance of activities to include valued activities Involve parents and carers, if possible Support development of autonomy
Services hard to access	Brief BA is relatively simple and quick to learn More professionals can learn to deliver Brief BA safely and well Structured worksheets to support therapist and young person
Problems with engagement	Focus on building therapeutic alliance Collaboration between young person and therapist Help the young person to identify 'what matters to *you*'
Cognitive problems	Keep it simple (but recognize it is not easy) Reduce demands on working memory Give written information and pictures and figures
Hopelessness	Therapy is time-limited – it instills hope and expectation that things can change Identify what a young person values – what matters to them? Increase valued activities Maximize rewards (including therapist reinforcement)
Motivation problems	Therapist provides as much positive reinforcement as possible Link activities to values Engage supporters

In Brief BA, we draw on two over arching theories: the *therapeutic alliance* and *behavioural theory*. It is very important that all therapists who use Brief BA understand these and can follow their principles. You may already be familiar with these theories; if you are not, don't worry because we will describe both of these in Chapter 10, and explain how they are essential when you treat young people with depression.

It is important to be aware that the therapeutic alliance is necessary in every part of therapy, from the beginning through to the end. It can change across therapy, and we will show you how to monitor the alliance at every session to make sure things don't go off track.

We discuss behavioural theory and the behavioural theory of depression in Chapter 11 and in relation to values and depression in Chapter 12. The behavioural theory of depression is a well-established, well-evidenced and relatively simple theory of what triggers depression, and, more importantly for therapists and young people, what keeps it going. If depression did not keep going we could just wait a while and things would get better. But they don't, so it is what keeps depression going that we directly tackle in Brief BA.

CHAPTER 10

Getting to Know the Young Person and Keeping Them Safe

The priority in any psychological therapy is to engage the young person and to keep them safe. No treatment can be helpful if the young person does not come to sessions and does not engage with the aims and rationale of therapy. Suicidal thoughts are a symptom of depression – in recent research, 60 per cent of young people with depression reported current active thoughts of suicide (Goodyer *et al.* 2017). Self-harm is also common among young people with depression and is a significant predictor of subsequent suicide attempts. Most alarmingly, rates of suicide among young women and young men rose significantly in the UK between 2012 and 2018. For these reasons, Brief BA includes a specific focus on engagement, building a therapeutic alliance with the young person and identifying and managing risk. In this chapter, we focus on the two key tasks of early sessions with the young person: 'Getting to know your client' and 'Keeping the young person safe'.

Getting to know your client

The therapeutic alliance

The therapeutic alliance refers to the relationship that develops between a therapist and client. In Brief BA, the therapeutic alliance is the foundation on which we build behavioural change and overcome symptoms of depression. In a good therapeutic alliance the client feels able to share information that is personal and may make them feel embarrassed or even ashamed. Ideally, they will feel able to discuss matters that they do not freely talk about anywhere else, and feel heard and understood. The therapist aims to provide an atmosphere that feels comfortable, unthreatening and 'safe'.

Some therapists and researchers (e.g. Horvath and Luborsky 1993; Rogers 1951) have argued that the therapeutic alliance between a therapist and their client (or the therapeutic relationship) is the key ingredient of therapy, and that a good therapeutic alliance is all that is needed for the client to benefit from psychotherapy. In other words, they think that the therapeutic alliance is 'necessary and sufficient' for change. However, we don't quite agree with that position.

There is extensive and consistent evidence that having a positive therapeutic alliance is significantly correlated with outcome in therapy. Clients who have a stronger or better alliance with their therapist tend to report more change at the end of therapy than those who have a less strong alliance. This is found across different types and 'schools' of psychotherapy (Fluckiger *et al.* 2018), and with adults as well as with children and young people (Karver *et al.* 2018). However, a significant correlation between alliance and treatment outcome does not mean that the therapeutic alliance *causes* change, or that an alliance, on its own, is enough for change to occur. Anyone with training in statistics or logic will be aware that correlation does not equal causation.

However, we do think that the therapeutic alliance is *necessary* for therapy to work. If a depressed young person doesn't feel supported, understood and listened to, and if they don't trust you, they probably won't come to the next session. If they don't come to the session, they can't benefit from therapy. So, if a depressed young person is to benefit from therapy, you need them to come back to the next session, and the one after that. The young person needs to be in the room. If they find it hard to be motivated and lack energy, the positive relationship with their therapist can help overcome their inertia. This is why building a therapeutic alliance with your client is your first and most important job.

Sometimes even when you have a really good therapeutic alliance your client doesn't come back for the next session. Our colleagues (O'Keeffe *et al.* 2019) have studied why young people 'drop out' of therapy. They found that some young people don't come back because they have started to feel better and don't want any more sessions. That's a good outcome for them, but frustrating for their therapist who may never find out how they did. Other young people have such difficult and chaotic lives that they can't get to the next session. That's not a good outcome, and we'd really like to be able to keep those young people in treatment and provide the support they need. A third group of young people stop coming to therapy, not because they feel better, or because they can't, but because they just don't rate their therapist or what is being offered. They choose to drop out of therapy. So, building a good therapeutic alliance with the young person may not guarantee successful treatment, but it definitely helps young people feel connected with the therapist, to want to come back to the next session, and to believe that their therapist can help them change.

What makes a good therapeutic alliance?

We think that Carl Rogers had it about right. He argued that all psychological therapists needed to offer their client three things. These were (and still are):

- Empathy
- Unconditional positive regard
- Congruence.

One great thing about Carl Rogers, and perhaps the most important reason that he is a legend in psychology, is that he didn't just argue that warmth, empathy and positive regard needed to be offered by therapists; Carl Rogers was the first psychologist to make a scientific study of psychotherapy (Goldfried 2007; Rogers 1965). He defined 'empathy', 'positive regard' and 'congruence' as follows:

- Empathy: The key characteristic of empathy is understanding another person's subjective reality as they experience it at any given moment. This requires an orientation toward the client's concerns and values that are relevant to them in that moment. In other words, empathy is the experience of trying to fully understand another person's world. Empathy is demonstrated through the therapist's attention and listening, using techniques such as reflection, paraphrasing and testing understanding. Through the use of empathy, the young person is able to experience a sense of being carefully listened to and understood.
- Unconditional positive regard: This concept incorporates acceptance, warmth, prizing and respect (Bozarth 2002). Gillon (2007) argued that the term 'positive' is used deliberately to

indicate the warm nature of the experience, rather than a cold form of passive acceptance indicating 'neutral passivity'. Through their positive regard for the young person, the therapist offers a compassionate and non-judgemental approach, and demonstrates that the young person is valued.

- Congruence: This refers to the therapist's capacity to be aware of their own experiences. This enables them to behave in a genuine, authentic and coherent way with the young person, rather than, for example, presenting themselves mainly in terms of their professional role.

Empathy, positive regard and congruence are the cornerstones of a good therapeutic alliance. However, these essential aspects of a good relationship do not capture everything that goes on in a therapeutic alliance. Both the therapist and the client want something to change; they are there to get something done. For this reason, the therapeutic alliance is also sometimes called the working alliance (Bordin 1979).

There are three core elements of a working alliance:

- The bond between the therapist and client
- The goals that they agree to work towards
- The tasks that they each perform to achieve those goals.

We like this way of thinking about the relationship between the therapist and their client. It highlights the fact that this is a partnership and that it is active and has a purpose. The therapist and their client both have work to do. These parts of a working alliance also directly map onto the practical aspects of Brief BA in terms of getting to know the young person, setting treatment goals and working towards these (as outlined in Part 2).

Is our therapeutic alliance okay?

Because the therapeutic relationship is such an essential part of treatment with a depressed young person, we strongly recommend that you use a systematic way of checking in with the young person and checking that their experience of treatment is positive. It can be difficult for young people to tell an adult that things are not okay. In our work we ask the young person to complete the simple and very brief Session Rating Scale (SRS; Duncan *et al.* 2003) at every session. This means that each and every session the young person is able to let you know how things are going for them, and gives you the opportunity to spot difficulties promptly, and to take action if necessary. As with all Routine Outcome Measures (ROMs), it is important to make sure that the young person knows that you check them each week and you will want to ask them about any concerns they have.

Using Routine Outcome Measures in Brief BA

Another way we can get to know the young person in Brief BA is through using ROMs. Depression in young people can be dangerous and hard to treat. In routine community Child and Adolescent Mental Health services, around a quarter of young people get worse, not better (Warren *et al.* 2010). Therefore, in Brief BA we want to keep a close eye on how the young person is feeling, if their symptoms are improving, getting worse or staying the same, if our therapeutic alliance is strong, and if there is any risk of self-harm or suicide. These are a lot of different things to monitor and it is easy to forget, or to misinterpret things and get things wrong.

Healthcare staff frequently misinterpret important information, and there is evidence that they also have a strong positive bias about their own performance. For example, much like car drivers, therapists routinely over-estimate their level of skill. Walfish, McAllister, O'Donnell and Lambert (2012) reported that 25 per cent of therapists rated their skills as in the top 10 per cent of therapists – and no therapists at all rated themselves as being below average as a therapist. Perhaps it is not surprising that therapists tend to hold inaccurate and overly positive views of their own skills – or at least they tell researchers that they are more than averagely skilful. But this is concerning because if we think we are better therapists than we are, it may mean that we are less concerned about improving, and less self-critical, and thus this interferes with learning and improving.

In Brief BA, it is important that therapists are reflective, examine their performance and try to be accurate in assessing their skills. This is because we have also found that therapists who have a more accurate judgement about their strengths and weaknesses are more competent, and those who think they are better therapists than they actually are, are, in fact, less competent (Brosan, Reynolds and Moore 2008). It is natural for new and trainee therapists to wonder if they are 'good enough'. We all worry about making mistakes and getting things wrong. Having supportive and constructive supervision and using self-reflection helps build our skills and our confidence. However, it is important to remain self-reflective after your initial period of training and to continue to use self-reflection to further improve your therapeutic skills. This is why we recommend that self-reflection becomes part of your routine clinical practice. Regular supervision and using information from ROMs with your client can help support this practice.

ROMs also help clinicians to monitor if a young person is feeling better or worse, if they have thoughts of suicide or self-harm, and if they are well engaged in treatment and with the therapist. For this reason, we strongly recommend that you use ROMs at every session, review them with the young person every time, use them to help you and the young person decide what to focus on in treatment, and bring them to and review them in supervision.

ROMs are used in a wide range of different health and medical contexts. They offer a quick and simple way to check key signs that the patient is okay, or is not okay. If you have a new baby, the nurse or health visitor will weigh them and measure them at every appointment. If you have surgery, a nurse will regularly and frequently check your breathing rate and your pulse. They are using ROMs. Patient-reported outcome measures (PROMs) are also used in a range of medical, surgical, community and mental health settings to assess patients' quality of life, symptoms (e.g. pain) and wellbeing. PROMs can help patients and healthcare professionals identify improvement and deterioration, help them communicate about the effects of treatment and make informed decisions about treatment and care, and they support collaboration between patients and healthcare staff.

Another important use of PROMs is that they can be used, across a service or across a group of patients, to indicate how well the service is working to improve patient wellbeing, or how that group of patients (e.g. from a particular local community or culture) respond to the treatment they are being offered. A major advantage of using PROMs at every session is that every patient or service user can be included in the data – if we only measure change at the start and end of treatment, any patient who does not attend the final session of treatment cannot be included in the data. These people are often the ones we want to know about most, to understand why they may not have finished the treatment.

Some researchers, clinicians and policy-makers argue that using PROMs increases treatment effectiveness, treatment efficiency and collaboration between clinicians and young people (e.g. Edbrooke-Childs, Wolport and Deighton 2016). This seems logical; after all, if we are able to use ROMs to intervene promptly when things are not going well, this should lead to better outcomes from treatment. Similarly, if we always discuss how things are going with our clients, and involve them in decisions that we make about their treatment in a systematic and sensitive way, this, surely, should improve collaboration between us. Surprisingly, however, the evidence to support these hypotheses is not very strong or of very good quality. There is some limited evidence that using PROMs in psychological therapies may improve effectiveness. For example, in a systematic review of 32 studies by Gondek *et al.* (2016), more than 50 per cent of studies reported that using PROMs resulted in significantly higher treatment effectiveness on at least one of the measures used. Putting this the other way, almost 50 per cent of studies did not show that using PROMs improved treatment effectiveness on any of the measures used. Another review of the use of PROMs in treatment of common mental health problems in adults found that across 12 studies and 3696 participants, there was insufficient evidence that using PROMs improved patient outcomes, and that the quality of the research was low (Kendrick *et al.* 2016).

In Brief BA, we use PROMs at the start and end of treatment and at every session (because not all young people seeking help with depression symptoms would refer to themselves as patients, we call these ROMs rather than PROMs). This helps us get to know the young person better, and to check how they are today, right now, in this room. The ROMs that we use include a question about self-harm and suicide; this means that every time we see them, the young person is always prompted to tell us if they have had these thoughts or behaved in a risky way, and neither they nor the therapist avoid the important question. If the young person indicates that they have had any self-harm or thoughts of suicide, then the priority for the therapist at that session is to assess the risk to the young person and to make sure that they can be kept safe.

Young people tell us that they find it helpful to review how they are doing each session, and at the end of treatment when they can compare how they feel now to how they felt at the start of treatment. We also always use ROMs in supervision with trainees and qualified clinicians. We review how each young person is doing in Brief BA and particularly focus on any young people who are not getting better, or who seem to be getting worse. This gives us an opportunity to review Brief BA, to ask if this is the best treatment for this young person now, and to consider putting in place alternatives, including referral on to a more specialist mental health service.

What Routine Outcome Measures should I use?

Most Child and Adolescent Mental Health services in England and many other countries already use a standard set of ROMs. If this is the case in your service, then you will not need to worry about this question. If you are not working in an English NHS Child and Adolescent Mental Health service and are interested in using the ROMs recommended for use in English Child and Adolescent Mental Health services, you can find them on the Child Outcomes Research Consortium (CORC).[1]

When selecting which ROM to use in your own clinical practice, there are a number of criteria that are important to bear in mind:

- Speed and brevity – the young person should be able to complete the session-by-session ROMs in five minutes or less
- Relevance – ROMs should have been developed and designed to assess the key difficulty that the young person presents with and you are working on together

1 www.corc.uk.net

- Validity – ROMs should measure what they say they measure for the type of client in front of you
- Sensitivity – ROMs should be able to pick up on small change, from session to session
- Interpretability – you and the young person should be able to quickly work out what their score on the measure means – how it compares to others (the norms) and if it has changed (better or worse)
- Flexibility – ideally, the ROM should be available in different languages or be simple enough to be adapted or translated for non-native speakers or young people who are not literate.

Keeping the young person safe

Using Brief BA in the treatment of adolescent depression involves an explicit and routine enquiry into the young person's thoughts and actions relating to self-harm and suicide.

This is an area of clinical work that many therapists find challenging and sometimes frightening. Other professionals (e.g. teachers, family doctors and school nurses) as well as parents are also often too anxious and worried to ask young people if they have any thoughts or plans to harm themselves. Attitudes towards people who self-harm can also be negative (Saunders *et al.* 2012). Many young people who do have thoughts or plans about suicide, or who have self-harmed or plan to self-harm, are therefore not given an opportunity to discuss this with anyone.

Because suicide is one of the leading causes of death among young people (ONS 2016), and because self-harm is a strong predictor of suicide (Morgan *et al.* 2017), both should be identified when present, and support and strategies introduced to keep the young person safe. The World Health Organization (WHO) recommends that all young people over 10 years old who have been identified with a mental health disorder, or who have experienced loss, interpersonal conflict or a severe life event should be asked about thoughts and plans to self-harm. In Brief BA, we use ROMs at every session to help identify (and then deal with) self-harm and suicidal thoughts, plans and behaviours.

Self-harm

Self-harm is not uniquely associated with depression, and is not always associated with suicidal thoughts and plans. However, it is one of the strongest predictors of suicide, and should therefore always be treated seriously. Self-harm refers to any kind of self-injury or self-poisoning.

Rates of self-harm vary across countries. In a transnational survey of 45,806 15- to 16-year-olds living in 17 European countries, Kokkevi *et al.* (2012) reported that the median rate of self-harm was 30.9 per cent, with 4.8 per cent harming themselves more than five times. Rates of self-harm were somewhat higher in the UK, where of 2179 young people, 36.8 per cent reported that they had self-harmed at least once and 8.5 per cent reported that they had harmed themselves more than five times. The risk factors for self-harm closely overlap with those for depression in young people, and include death of a parent, sexual or physical abuse, family conflict and deprivation. Age is also a predictor, with the incidence of self-harm increasing significantly after the age of 12 (Fox *et al.* 2015).

The reasons for self-harm in young people are not well understood. Some young people report that hurting or harming themselves helps them to regulate very strong and unpleasant emotions. Sometimes after completing the act of self-harm young people describe experiencing a feeling of relief. Self-harm is linked to impulsivity and impaired decision-making (McHugh *et al.* 2019). Young people who are overwhelmed by strong confusing and unpleasant emotions, or who have overwhelming practical difficulties, may find that self-harm offers brief but immediate reinforcement. This reinforcement therefore makes it more likely that they will use self-harm again as a coping strategy, especially if they find it hard to inhibit impulses.

Self-harm elicits very strong emotions in other people, including therapists and other professionals. Family members report feeling shocked, angry and disbelieving (Ferrey *et al.* 2016). Young people report trying to avoid seeking emergency medical attention because of perceived stigma and punitive responses from emergency healthcare staff (Owens *et al.* 2016). Ironically, these negative responses from professionals towards young people who self-harm can further exacerbate their negative self-evaluation and feelings of shame, and tend to increase their risk of repeating self-harm. Given this evidence, it is clearly essential that all clinicians working with young people who self-harm treat them with compassionate and non-discriminatory care. As a Brief BA therapist, your positive and collaborative therapeutic alliance with the young person is an important way to minimize any negative impacts of disclosing self-harm, and to encourage young people to share difficult information with you.

Suicidal thoughts and suicidal intent among young people

Thinking about suicide, either actively (e.g. 'I want to kill myself') or passively (e.g. 'The world would be better off without me') is one of the symptoms used to diagnose depression in adolescents and adults. Not surprisingly, therefore, suicidal thoughts are quite common among depressed young people. For example, a treatment study with 465 depressed young people who were assessed using a structured clinical interview (Goodyer *et al.* 2017) found that 61 per cent of the participants reported active thoughts of suicide and over one-third (34 per cent) had attempted suicide at some point in their lifetime. For this reason, suicidal thoughts and attempts are always of concern when working with young people who are depressed.

Suicide attempts are also fairly common in the wider adolescent population. Kokkevi and colleagues (2012) asked over 45,000 young people from 17 different countries if they had ever tried to kill themselves. Across all countries involved, 10.5 per cent of 15- to 16-year-olds had attempted suicide at least one time, and 4.8 per cent had tried more than once. In the UK the corresponding rates of suicide attempt and repeated suicide attempts were similar, at 9.2 per cent and 4 per cent of participants.

Fortunately, completed suicide is still uncommon among young people. In the UK, in 2018, there were 5.8 deaths per 100,000 young people aged 15 to 19 (ONS 2019). Suicide remains, however, a leading cause of death in this otherwise usually healthy age group. In a case review of the 145 young people who died by suicide in England between January 2014 and April 2015, a number of issues appeared to be common in the months before the death. These included academic pressure, bullying, bereavement, suicide by a family member or friend, use of drugs or excessive alcohol, physical health problems and family conflict. Almost half of the young people who died by suicide had had no previous involvement with mental health services (Rodway *et al.* 2016).

Suicide is very hard to predict (Sedgwick and Ougrin 2019), and for this reason it is essential that young people who are at increased risk of suicide, including young people who are being treated for depression, are actively monitored. To reduce the burden on therapists and to make sure that young people always have an opportunity to talk about any suicidal thoughts they have, we always ask about suicidal thoughts or plans, as well as self-harm, at every session. Making this routine and standardized means that the question becomes less emotionally loaded, and conveys the message that it is always okay to talk to the therapist about suicide and self-harm (Mathias *et al.* 2012).

CHAPTER 11

Rewards and Reinforcement

The Behavioural Theory of Depression

In this chapter, we focus on the core theory of Brief BA – behavioural theory. Behavioural theory is familiar to all students of psychology, and suggests that our actions and behaviour are shaped by their consequences. The rewards and punishments that follow our behaviours make it more or less likely that we will repeat them. Therefore, although we usually associate depression with emotions and feelings, the behavioural treatment of depression focuses on changing key behaviours that keep depression going and interfere with recovery.

Behavioural theory

Brief BA for depression builds on a very well-established theory that has decades of supporting research and evidence. *Operant conditioning* was first described by Skinner (1938) to explain how animals and humans learn. At its most simple, the theory of operant conditioning proposes that if we are rewarded (or reinforced) for a behaviour, we are likely to repeat it. The behaviour that was reinforced is *strengthened*. Conversely, if we are punished for a behaviour, we are less likely to do it again and the behaviour is *weakened*. There are two types of reinforcement and reward, and these are central to how we use BA.

Table 11.1. Operant conditioning – the effects of reinforcement and punishment

	Reinforcement	Punishment
Add something	Positive reinforcement, e.g. give money, sweets Behaviour more likely to be repeated	Positive punishment, e.g. give a smack Behaviour less likely to be repeated
Remove something	Negative reinforcement, e.g. avoid a smack Behaviour more likely to be repeated	Negative punishment, e.g. take away money, sweets Behaviour less likely to be repeated

Positive reinforcement is when, following a behaviour, we receive or experience something desirable or enjoyable. Most of us experience positive reinforcement or rewards many times every day. For example, we are positively reinforced when we feel good after going for run, watching a sunset, enjoying a meal, when we receive praise or affection, feel satisfied after working hard or feel close to someone. Positive reinforcement or reward makes us feel good, encourages us to repeat the behaviour, and helps us get more out of life. Parents often use positive reinforcement to help their children learn new behaviours – for example, they reward them when they sleep in their own bed.

Positive reinforcement can be extrinsic or intrinsic. For example, when we go to work we receive an extrinsic reward – our pay. Work can also provide many intrinsic rewards. These include enjoyment of work tasks in and of themselves, social rewards – for example laughing with our work colleagues or feeling part of a team – and achievement-related rewards, for example when we complete a task, reach a goal or overcome a challenge.

Negative reinforcement is when something unwanted or disliked is removed, stops, is taken away or avoided. Negative reinforcement affects how we behave every day in a range of situations. It is widely used to make sure we follow rules and regulations. For example, we drive at or under the speed limit to make sure we do not get a speeding ticket and a fine. We plan a journey to work or to an appointment to make sure we arrive on time and do not have the embarrassment (or worse) and anxiety associated with arriving late.

Negative reinforcement also has an important role in maintaining behaviours associated with avoidance. For example, imagine that I am 14 years old. I am invited to go out and meet some teenagers I don't know. I feel pretty shy and 'know' that I won't be able to join in and that the others will think I'm stupid. I make up a reason not to go and immediately feel relieved.

This feeling of relief (reward) is negative reinforcement. I decide to stay at home instead of going out to meet new people. This avoidant behaviour has been negatively reinforced. This means that next time I have the opportunity to avoid a similar social situation I am more likely to decide to stay at home and avoid it. Negative reinforcement therefore makes us feel better immediately. However, negative reinforcement increases the chance that we will avoid the same situation or scary thing the next time we experience it. The difficulty with this is that in the long term it reduces the opportunities for positive reinforcement that can be gained from such scenarios (e.g. having fun, making new friends) and may also reduce the likelihood of other sources of positive reinforcement (e.g. friends stop inviting you to parties, stop 'liking' you on social media).

Punishment leads to behaviours being less likely to be repeated. *Positive punishment* is given when a behaviour is followed by a negative consequence. Punishment is widely used in daily life to shape our behaviours. For example, when driving we may be punished with a fine if we exceed the speed limit. Punishments include physical reprimands such as smacking or hitting, and verbal reprimands, for example being told off or being given a verbal warning. *Negative punishment* involves the removal or deprivation of rewards. A child may be forbidden to play on their computer or be sent to bed early.

The behavioural theory of depression

The behavioural theory of depression (Ramnerö, Folke and Kanter 2016) proposes that different mechanisms are responsible for the initial onset of depression and for the maintenance of depression and low mood.

The initial onset of depression

According to the behavioural theory, depression is triggered by an event that leads to a reduction in *positive reinforcement*. Young people experience two main types of events that trigger depression (Clark and Oates 1995; Goodyer *et al.* 2000). The first involves a break in a relationship, including breaking up with a boyfriend or girlfriend, arguing with friends, siblings moving home, parental divorce or separation, bereavement, separation from siblings or friends, and bullying or abuse. Each of these life events is associated with loss and with a reduction in positive reinforcement or rewards. The second type of events that trigger depression and depression symptoms are also often experienced by young people and are linked to achievement and failure. These include failing an exam, losing a job, or not being picked for a football team. Here, reinforcement and rewards associated with status, money or achievement of important goals are lost.

Imagine Tom, aged 15.

> Tom is a very keen hockey player. He plays for the school team and for a local team at weekends. His school team are well respected and this year their aim is to win the county championship. Many of his friends also play hockey, and this means that lots of his social life is based around hockey.
>
> In November, Tom is injured. He has a broken leg and this means that he cannot play hockey again for the rest of the season.
>
> The immediate impact of the accident is that Tom has to spend a week at home before he goes back to school. His family are very caring, his friends come to visit him after school, and he even gets a 'Get Well' card from his whole class. He can spend the day at home playing on the computer and doesn't get set any homework or have to do any schoolwork.
>
> After a couple of days, Tom is bored and lonely. He is spending a lot of time on his own and misses his friends. He can't get up and go out and take exercise, and feels sluggish and irritable. He is annoyed with himself for having had the accident and begins to realize that he won't be able to play hockey again for months! His parents notice that he is a bit down – they think this is understandable and try to cheer him up, bring him new books and games and try to get him interested in planning the family holiday. His girlfriend Eva comes round every night after school and he looks forward to seeing her and hearing about everything that's going on.

During this period Tom has lost a number of different types of positive reinforcement – social reinforcement from seeing his friends at school every day, physical exercise because he is immobile, and feelings of achievement that he gets when he plays hockey, especially if his team win. His family have given him a lot of positive reinforcement, especially when they notice he is a bit upset or sad, or just quiet. His girlfriend is making a special effort to cheer him up. Everyone, including Tom, thinks that what he is feeling is completely understandable.

> After a week Tom goes back to school. His leg is in a plaster cast and so he is able to move around, but slowly and with a lot of effort – it hurts to move much. He can't manage to get the bus to school so his dad drops him off in the morning and he gets a lift home from another parent from school. His parents are relieved to see him go back so quickly. Everyone at school is really pleased to see him back at school and his plaster cast is very quickly covered in cartoons, signatures and a few rude images. Tom settles down back at school and starts to try to catch up on the work he has missed.

Lewinsohn (1974) and Beck (1983) suggested that loss of *positive reinforcement* leads to depression if the individual is not able to replace the lost source of reinforcement with an alternative. For example, if a young person loses a friendship or group of friends, the lost positive reinforcement could, in theory, be replaced if they made new friends or focused on an alternative source of reinforcement. The impact of failing an exam need not lead to depression if the young person is able to retake the exam or has other more notable or important achievements. Lewinsohn also suggested that during this initial onset period, some individuals also receive positive reinforcement for depressed behaviour if their family and friends increase attention or give them more social support than usual. This is certainly what happened to Tom – he lost a lot of *positive reinforcement* (friends, sport, physical activity), but his family provided some new sources of reinforcement by being caring and concerned about him.

Maintaining depression and depressive symptoms

Bad things happen to us all. However, most people who experience a negative event do not develop sustained periods of depression and low mood. It is important to understand why depression keeps going.

The behavioural theory of depression suggests that depression is maintained, or keeps going, because of negative reinforcement or avoidance. As discussed above, *negative reinforcement* has short-term benefits and removes discomfort, anxiety or other negative emotions that we predict or expect. However, this initial reward (the feeling of relief) is short-lived, and negative reinforcement has unexpected negative consequences for the young person.

Let's consider Tom again.

> Tom returns to school after a week off at home. His friends and teachers are pleased to see him. His leg will recover and everyone expects that he will be able play hockey again next season.
>
> Tom is really pleased to be back at school and able to spend time with his friends. However, because of his broken leg there are lots of things he still cannot do. He is not able to attend or take part in training sessions after school or at the weekend, and he obviously cannot play in any matches. He is also not able to be independent – he can't get the bus on his own and so relies on other people to drive him everywhere, including school.
>
> Many of Tom's friends are in the hockey team. Two evenings in the week and at the weekend he misses the training sessions and the matches. At school he hears his friends talking about the match they lost, the goals that they scored (and missed) and the jokes they had on the bus on their way to the match.
>
> Tom tries to keep in with his friends, but after a few weeks he feels like a spare part. Tom's friends try to help him feel involved by telling him about each match but this makes him feel more left out. He doesn't want to hear about the last match, see any pictures or match reports on social media, or to talk about tactics for the next match. Tom feels that he has nothing to contribute to the group. He also can't join in any physical activities, and because he has to spend a lot of time sitting down, he can't even just hang out with his friends in the park.

During this period Tom is still missing out on a lot of positive reinforcement. Although his family and girlfriend are supportive and caring, this doesn't replace the sense of achievement and fun he had playing hockey and the laughs and jokes he had with his friends. He has lost a lot of independence and the rewards associated with making decisions for himself.

> Every Christmas, Tom looks forward to the hockey club Christmas party. Parents and friends are invited and all the team members receive prizes for their role in the team. This year, as the date for the party approaches, Tom realizes that he doesn't want to go. How can he enjoy it as usual? He will feel left out and embarrassed. On the day before the party, Tom has a slight headache and a cough. It's nothing serious, but he realizes that if he isn't feeling well he can avoid going to the party and feeling like a spare part. His parents will understand and no one will make a fuss.
>
> Tom misses the party. He stays at home with his parents and girlfriend, and they all get a pizza and go to the cinema together. It's not such a bad evening, and Tom is relieved that he didn't have to go and sit through the party, watching everyone else have a great time.

Missing the hockey Christmas party leads to Tom receiving both positive *and* negative reinforcement:

- *Positive reinforcement* – attention from his family and girlfriend, pizza, a trip to the cinema

- *Negative reinforcement* – the feeling of relief that he experienced as a result of avoiding the party.

Next week at school Tom hears everyone laughing and joking about the prize giving. He thinks he did the right thing – it would have been really embarrassing to be given a prize when he's not even in the team at the moment. But he also feels more left out. His friends are all excited about other Christmas parties. Tom realizes that he doesn't want to go to any of the other parties either. He doesn't want to have to sit down while other people are dancing and messing about, he doesn't want to tell people about his accident, and he knows that he won't be able to just relax and have a good time.

Tom has a quiet Christmas at home with his family. His parents try to cheer him up with his favourite food and drinks. He feels a bit suffocated and gets irritated by their attention. Tom starts staying up late playing computer games and waking up later and later each day. He eats a lot of junk food and misses meals with his family. His girlfriend visits and they hang out a few times but she has a lot of parties to go to and her own family to spend time with. It's hard to know what to talk about. Tom finds himself spending more time alone. He plays on his computer, listens to music in his room, and checks out social media to find out what his friends are doing.

By the time Tom goes back to school in January he feels very isolated. His cast is removed and he starts physiotherapy. He notices that he has put on some weight and feels really unfit. Everything is a huge effort and he just can't be bothered with it all. Everyone is getting prepared for the big exams in the summer and Tom still hasn't caught up with the work he missed in November. He starts to spend more time trying to catch up and doing his homework, but feels he is falling further and further behind. He can't concentrate and feels stupid. Tom can't help comparing himself to his friends who all seem to be having so much fun. He doesn't think he fits in with them any more. At school he tries to avoid them and spends break time in the library.

By January, two months after he had his accident, Tom's leg is definitely much better. With physiotherapy over the next few months he will probably be able to play hockey again next season. However, Tom is beginning to get stuck in a negative cycle. His sleep and eating patterns have changed. He feels a failure, fat, unfit, stupid, isolated and lonely.

Tom now behaves very differently. He is caught in a negative cycle of depression. This keeps going because of two distinct but related factors:

- *Negative reinforcement* – Tom's behaviour of avoiding activities, people and events creates negative reinforcement. This initially makes him feel better as he doesn't have to do things that he thinks he will find difficult. Unfortunately, however, avoiding social activities, his friends and other events that are important to him also means that he becomes more isolated and more distant from his friends

- *Positive reinforcement* – because Tom is avoiding things and isolating himself, he now gets far less positive reinforcement. As a result, he gets much less out of life and his life lacks the 'feel-good factor'. The lack of positive reinforcement and 'feel-good factor' further lowers his mood, motivation and energy levels, and this makes it more difficult for him to engage in activities. Opportunities for positive reinforcement reduce even further.

This is the key cycle that we use in Brief BA to explain depression to young people and their parents (see Figure 11.1). Although every young person experiences depression in their own unique way, this simple cycle captures the important shared experiences and explains why they are feeling depressed, low or lacking enjoyment, and also importantly, why they find it so hard to change.

Brief BA treatment of adolescent depression

The behavioural theory of depression helps us understand how young people become depressed and why they remain depressed. Importantly, it can also be used to structure a psychological therapy to treat depression. The treatment of depression is based on the idea that depression is maintained by lack of *positive reinforcement* and sustained *negative reinforcement* and avoidance. To reverse this cycle, in Brief BA we aim to increase *positive reinforcement* (rewards) and reduce *negative reinforcement* and avoidance.

Brief BA focuses on why depression is maintained or keeps going. Although we can often identify specific triggers, these are now in the past. We cannot magic away Tom's broken leg or rewind the clock and help him go to those Christmas parties that he missed. But we can help him change what he is doing today, tomorrow and in the future.

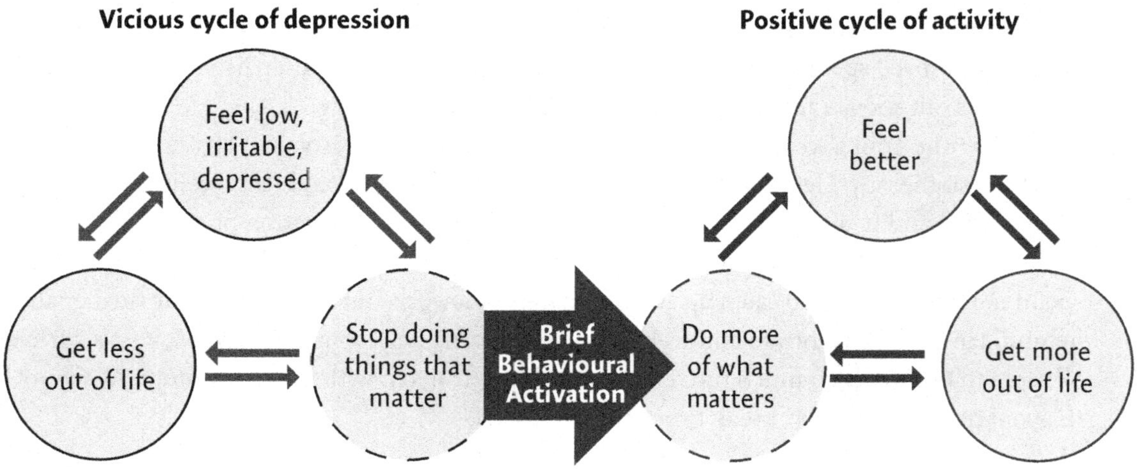

Figure 11.1. The Brief BA model

Psychoeducation

Psychoeducation is a key part of Brief BA, and has a number of important advantages:

- It gives the young person (and where possible, their parents or carers) a clear explanation of why they feel as they do (i.e. low, irritable, and/or not enjoying things) and why they cannot escape these negative feelings
- It normalizes and validates their feelings
- It helps young people understand that they are not alone in experiencing these symptoms and difficulties; others have similar problems
- It shows a possible way to break the cycle that they are stuck in
- The rationale for treatment is made clear and explicit
- The therapist and young person (and parent/s) share an understanding of depression
- It can help engagement, and builds collaboration and the therapeutic alliance
- It provides a clear way for parents or carers to support the young person.

In Brief BA, we explain what depression is and why it keeps going as soon as possible, ideally in Session 1. This is because young people and their parents usually want to understand why they are having difficulties. Whenever possible, we invite parents or carers to join part of Session 1 and describe the cycle of depression to them and their child together. Young people and their parents therefore know that they have been told the same information. We also reinforce this information in the worksheets that parents and young people are given so that they do not have to remember the information.

The Brief BA cycle of depression gives them a simple way to understand what keeps depression and low mood going, and why they have found it so difficult to change. We use diagrams and figures to help young people understand more easily (see Part 2). For example, we use Figure 11.1 to illustrate the negative cycle of depression (on the left) and how treatment will help change this into a positive cycle (on the right). To make the model directly relevant to the young person, we use their own words and experiences to fill in the negative cycle with them during the session. We check out that this matches their experience. Taking time to do this carefully with the young person is an important part of engaging them in treatment and building a positive therapeutic relationship. It may be the first time that anyone has explained depression to them.

So, working with Tom, we might agree:

'I feel stupid and lonely'

'So I spend a lot of time in my room' and

'I don't see my friends any more or play hockey.'

This means that,

'I get less out of life'

'Which then makes me feel even worse, more lonely and fed up.'

Using positive reinforcement to increase reward and reduce depression symptoms

In Brief BA, we treat depression by increasing the positive reinforcement and rewards that the young person receives for healthy, non-depressed behaviour. Positive reinforcement can be obtained in many different ways, and there are differences between people in what they find rewarding. This means that Brief BA is always tailored to each individual young person. To help identify activities that will be associated with potent rewards, we work with the young person's values, or what matters to them (see Chapter 10). When we know what matters most to the young person, we work with them to plan simple activities that relate to their values. Introducing *valued activities* leads to greater reward and positive reinforcement and to more positive mood. We use the therapeutic alliance and the young person's family and friends to support them in doing these activities. Wherever possible, we include valued activities within the therapy session, and then help the young person to decide what they will do between sessions.

In Brief BA, we also use positive reinforcement freely in our sessions. Reinforcement may be more effective and powerful if it is received immediately, especially for people with depression (Rehm and Plakosh 1975). We use behaviours to show that they value the young person. Smiling, nodding, paying attention and listening carefully are all positively reinforcing for most young people. These therapist behaviours also help build the therapeutic alliance. We also use positive reinforcement when the young person shows any signs of engaging in treatment and when they behave in any way that is non-depressed. Signs of engaging in treatment include attending sessions, talking in sessions, attempting tasks, for example monitoring their mood, completing ROMs and trying to behave in a non-depressed way, even if they still feel depressed.

Inside and outside the session, Brief BA therapists help the young person to get more positive reinforcement and reward by changing their behaviours in small but important ways. An important element of the behavioural treatment of depression is that rewarding activities are introduced gradually and in stages. Young people with depression are not optimistic about the chance of success. They usually feel hopeless, worthless and useless. Typically, they are not confident that treatment will help them and are frightened that it will not. It is important to pace behaviour changes carefully and to choose a behaviour change that is most rewarding. Therefore, we start with simple and small behavioural changes. In every session we look for opportunities to try out small behaviours that will reward the young person so that they experience positive reinforcement immediately and before they leave the session. Over several sessions we gradually build the complexity and demands of the valued activities that young people do between sessions. By the end of Brief BA the aim is that the young person is able to engage in a range of valued activities and that they consequently receive more positive reinforcement and more varied types of positive reinforcement.

Social learning theory

Operant conditioning theory is a powerful way to explain how humans learn and why they behave in the ways they do. The concepts of positive and negative reinforcement help explain why individuals become depressed and why they stay depressed, and provide the basis for a highly effective treatment for depression.

In Brief BA, we supplement the core theory of operant conditioning with social learning theory (Bandura 1978). This proposes that, in addition to learning as a result of rewards (and punishment), people learn from others, by observing, imitating and modelling. Bandura (1978) identified three types of modelling:

- Live models, where someone demonstrates the desired behaviour
- Verbal instruction, in which the desired behaviour is described
- Symbolic modelling, where learning occurs via some kind of indirect media (e.g. films, television, the internet).

We use social learning theory to help parents and other important adults to learn how to support their child to reduce their depression and build back healthy positive reinforcement. Although parents of adolescents with depression often want to support their son or daughter, they do not usually know how best to do this. In some families where there is a depressed adolescent, family members cope with difficulties through increasing control, conflict and/or avoidance (Kouros and Garber 2014; Stark *et al.* 1990). These behaviours contribute to a family environment in which parents find it difficult to give their child positive reinforcement. The family environment therefore contributes to their depression symptoms and lack of reward.

In Brief BA, when possible, parents or carers are invited to engage in therapy. This can be in different ways, depending on the context. Before treatment begins the parent is involved in the assessment, either in person or on the phone. Parents are given information – by hand, email or post – about Brief BA, as well as copies of the worksheets used in each session. Ideally, parents are invited to attend some treatment sessions, including the first and last sessions. When parents are not able to attend treatment sessions they are sent written material to explain Brief BA for adolescent depression.

When parents attend Brief BA sessions, live modelling and verbal information can show them how to make small but important changes. The therapist acts as a live model to the parent. They demonstrate how to increase positive reinforcement for the young person through praise, attention and other verbal and non-verbal behaviours. The parent observes how the therapist listens to the young person, and how they focus on reinforcing very small behaviours.

Social learning theory is a powerful way to change, often in a subtle way, an important part of the young person's environment and to extend the impact of Brief BA into their everyday life – at home. However, it is also important to recognize the context in which many young people and their families live. Young people with depression and their parents share multiple risk factors for depression including their environment (e.g. income level, housing, education), shared negative life events (e.g. parental divorce or separation, unemployment, house relocation) and genetics. Parents, as well as their children, are therefore at elevated risk of depression (Guffanti *et al.* 2016). If parents who have a depressed teenager are also experiencing depression or other mental health problems, or adverse living conditions or chronic adversity, it is very challenging for them to provide positive reinforcement and to support their child to overcome depression symptoms. It is therefore likely to be useful to the young person if their parent is able to access evidence-based treatment for their own difficulties, as well as any available sources of practical and social support. Brief BA therapists can often be sources of signposting or direct referral to such services for the parents of the young people they work with.

CHAPTER 12

Why 'What Matters to You' is Important

One of the key characteristics of Brief BA is that it emphasizes the importance of 'valued activities'. Identifying the young person's *values* (i.e. *what matters to them)* helps deepen our relationship with the young person and get to know them even better. Identifying what matters to them, distinct from what matters to their friends, family and wider social group, is an important part of building their identity. Understanding what really matters to the young person is also a key step towards helping them increase *positive reinforcement*, which will be more intrinsically rewarding to them and increase the 'feel-good factor'.

What are values?

When we talk about values in Brief BA with young people we tend to refer to 'what matters to you?' This way of describing values is clear and straightforward, and most young people understand it easily. A good metaphor for values is a 'compass' that helps guide the direction of our behaviours. In an ethical framework, 'values' are individual beliefs that motivate people to act one way or another.

Why do we focus on values in Brief BA for young people with depression?

We know that many young people who have depression are already active and busy, and that being active does not help them overcome depression. Therefore, simply adding further activities to their current schedules does not seem likely to help. The key to improving symptoms of depression is to increase activities that are positively reinforcing for the young person and which therefore increase their experience of reward.

There are a number of reasons for our focus on 'what matters to you?' Some of these relate to the nature of depression, and others are specific to the developmental period of adolescence. First let's consider why focusing on values is of particular relevance to young people.

Values are developmentally salient

As discussed in Chapter 9, adolescence is a critical period of development. It sets a trajectory for our wellbeing, aspirations, relationships and cognitions, emotions and behaviours throughout life. Because our thinking abilities improve quickly during this period, we are more able to step back and take a look at who we are, what kind of person we are and what kind of person we want to become, think about what we want from life, and plan for the future. Therefore, during adolescence our concept of 'who we are', that is, our 'self', becomes more relevant. It is influenced by our experiences and life events, including experiences of common mental health problems, such as depression. Over a number of years our concept of 'self' becomes more elaborated and consolidated during adolescence and early adulthood.

Our self-concept does not start to develop during adolescence. At around 18 months, infants begin to have a rudimentary sense of who they are and that they are distinct from other people. This is described as 'self-awareness'. By the age of three to four, children can describe themselves (i.e. 'me-self') in concrete terms (e.g. 'I am a girl'; Harter 2006). During early to middle childhood, children become increasingly able to evaluate themselves as either 'good' or 'bad'. However, during adolescence, cognitive development and the ability to engage in abstract thinking, self-reflection and social comparison support a dramatic increase in the complexity and sophistication of the 'self'. Adolescents can engage in more thoughtful and higher-order thinking about 'who they are' (Harter 2012). They also begin to understand that their image of themselves may differ according to the situation. New aspects of self-concept that involve different roles, relationships and associated perceptions emerge (e.g. self as a swimmer, friend, sister etc.). Thus, a key developmental task in late adolescence and early adulthood is to synthesize these different aspects and to develop a coherent sense of self (Damon and Hart 1988; Donahue *et al.* 1993; Harter 1998).

It is suggested that self-images are derived from our memories of personal experiences, or autobiographical memories (Conway 2005; Conway and Pleydell-Pearce 2000). Images of 'the self' that relate to adolescent experiences appear to have a lasting impact; when asked to remember important times in their life history, adults over the age of 40 disproportionately recall memories from between the ages of 15 to 30 (Rubin and Schulkind 1997; Rubin, Wetzler and Nebes 1986). This influence of adolescent and early adulthood experiences on the self and memory is referred to as the 'reminiscence bump'. Conway (2005) suggested that experiences recalled from this period might be 'self-defining' and reflect vivid, emotionally intense memories (Singer and Salovey 1993). Thus, adolescent self-images reflect an important pool of self-knowledge, which can last a lifetime.

Values, or 'what matters to me?', are closely related to our sense of who we are, or our 'self'. In childhood, values are absorbed from the social environment and learned directly from others (for example, parents, teachers, religious leaders) via direct instruction and modelling. During adolescence and young adulthood, our values continue to be shaped by family and teachers, but are increasingly influenced by peers and by exposure to other groups and social contexts (see Chapter 9). As we become more mature, values are likely to reflect a wider range of experiences and be modified by moral, religious and ethical beliefs. Values held by adults tend to be relatively stable over periods of ten years. During late childhood and adolescence, values are emerging, changing and developing, and are thus less stable. For example, Vecchione *et al.* (2019) found that between the ages of 10 and 12 young people endorsed more highly values related to openness to change and achievement and power. Other values (e.g. security and benevolence) were stable over the same time period.

In Brief BA, asking a young person 'what matters to you?' is almost always something that captures their attention and provokes interest. Some young people have already begun to think about this question and welcome the opportunity to share their thoughts and ideas. Others have not yet begun to consider it. For this group, being asked 'what matters to you?' and having that idea that they can have a separate and individual set of values, different from those held by their family, friends or teachers, is both novel and intriguing. Asking 'what matters to *you*?' also makes it explicit that their wishes and needs are what drives treatment, and this enhances and reinforces the collaboration between the young persona and the therapist.

Young people develop at different rates, and there is a vast difference in maturity between the average 12-year-old and the average 17-year-old, as well as significant variation between young people of the same chronological age. So thinking about 'what matters to you?' can be challenging. In addition, depression can impede cognitive functioning and interfere with abstract thinking and memory. In Brief BA, our aim is to make it as easy as possible to identify a young person's values, and so we provide key tools to help with this (see Chapter 4 and also Session 3).

Identifying values helps build a positive self-image

Negative self-perception is one of the ten symptoms that are part of the diagnostic criteria for depression in adolescents (DSM-5; APA 2013). It is also one of the most frequently observed symptoms of depression in young people (Orchard *et al.* 2017). Emerging evidence suggests that negative self-evaluation may also predict the severity of depression and the depression diagnostic status in young people (Orchard and Reynolds 2018).

There is consistent evidence that young people with depression hold negative views of their 'self'. For example, depressed adolescents endorsed more negative and fewer positive adjectives as self-referent (i.e. related to 'me') than healthy controls (Auerbach *et al.* 2015). Young people with elevated depression symptoms also endorsed negative adjectives more quickly, and positive adjectives more slowly, than adolescents who reported fewer symptoms of depression (Connolly, Abramson and Alloy 2016). In contrast, young people who are not depressed hold highly positive self-images. For example, Hards *et al.* (2019a) found that the most common self-images generated by young people included 'happy', 'funny', 'kind' and 'friendly'.

Focusing on 'what matters to you?' in Brief BA provides a way for the therapist and the young person to explore, in a non-threatening way, a range of different values and related to these more positive self-images. As shown in the worksheets (regarding life areas and values), we provide a simple structure to identify values. This has three columns:

- Me – hobbies/fun, looking after myself, physical health
- Things that matter – education/work, the things I need to do, the 'bigger picture'
- People who matter – family, friends, important other(s).

Young people we have worked with have expressed many different types of value, but they tend to find it much easier to initially identify values that relate to the final column, 'People who matter'. This is consistent with the evidence from neuroscience and developmental psychology that young people place very high priority on the relationships they have with other people, including their family. It is also consistent with research (e.g. Hards *et al.* 2019b; Orchard and Reynolds 2019) that shows that even when they were depressed, young people described themselves as 'friendly', 'helpful' and 'kind'. These positive pro-social self-images relating to 'people who matter' are an easy place to start discussing 'what matters to you?' with young people. They also immediately highlight important and positive aspects of their self-image and provide a range of valued activities that can be carried out.

It is also important and helpful to encourage the young person to identify other types of values. This helps their focus from being exclusively about themselves in relation to others. Values associated with their own wellbeing highlight that they are also important. It opens up the possibility of values linked to improving their fitness, diet and sleep. Identifying 'things that matter' highlights wider aspects of life, including, but not exclusively, their education and occupation. This provides an important link with young people's 'possible selves'.

'Possible selves' reflects the future-oriented part of the 'self'. They are based on the current self and reflect what an individual hopes, expects or fears to become in the future (Markus and Nurius 1986; Packard and Conway 2006). The ability to imagine the future is important and has many adaptive functions. These include improving motivation, that is, working towards future goals (Strauss, Griffin and Parker 2012), increasing problem-solving (Taylor *et al.* 1998) and self-regulation (Oyserman *et al.* 2004). Young people tend to be optimistic about their futures (Bohn and Berntsen 2013) in that they hold more positive and fewer negative possible selves (Wilson *et al.* 2012).

Some prominent theories of depression suggest that depressed individuals hold a negative view of the future (Beck 1979) and expect negative, aversive outcomes to occur in the future (Abramson, Metalsky and Alloy 1989). Horwitz *et al.* (2017) concluded that a lack of positive expectations about the future was a significant predictor of depression and suicidal behaviour in young people with elevated suicide risk. Similarly, Timbremont and Braet (2006) reported that a negative view of the future predicted depression severity one year later in a non-clinical sample of adolescents.

There is some evidence that using psychological interventions to develop a more positive future 'self' is associated with reduced symptoms in young people (e.g. McCay *et al.* 2006). This may be especially important for young people because both their current 'self' and their future possible 'self' is developing and presumably malleable (Knox *et al.* 1998). In Brief BA, we address the current 'self' and future 'possible self' through considering 'what matters to you?' Spending time identifying their values is also important because values can be implicit, or not in our conscious awareness. Having space and support to examine their personal values can help a young person to make important decisions about their future relationships, lifestyle, education and employment, and how to prioritize these.

Valued activities increase the power of positive reinforcement

The key change mechanism in Brief BA is increased positive reinforcement for non-depressed behaviour. To break the negative cycle of depression we need to help the young person get more out of life and experience the 'feel-good factor'. However, to do this we also need to overcome the barriers of low motivation, fatigue and anhedonia. This is a key challenge, both for therapists and for depressed young people.

Focusing on 'what matters to you?' provides different ways to increase positive reinforcement. First, asking the question and taking an interest in this key developmental area directly taps into a young person's identity and concerns. This focused interest is itself positively reinforcing and helps improve the therapeutic relationship and connection between the young person and the therapist.

Second, identifying the young person's values gives the therapist information about activities that are likely to be congruent with the young person and intrinsically motivating. This additional motivation can be helpful in overcoming the many barriers to change that depressed young people face. In discussing what matters to them with an interested adult they can demonstrate passion, commitment, concerns, confusion and conflict. All of these emotions help further engage the young person with the process of Brief BA, and help build their therapeutic alliance.

Third, identifying 'what matters to you?' means that the therapist and the young person can collaboratively start to plan activities that are important and more positively reinforcing. Therefore, by linking activities to values we can increase the amount of reward that the young person can receive from taking part in Brief BA. Because they receive more reward (positive reinforcement) from the activities they carry out, their mood improves more quickly. Positive reinforcement also means that the activity is more likely to be repeated.

CHAPTER 13

Brief BA Therapeutic Techniques and Strategies

Brief BA is based on the principles of behavioural theory and aims to overcome depression by increasing positive reinforcement and rewards. Depressed young people have a range of characteristics (see Chapter 9) that make it very difficult to engage in psychological therapy. Within Brief BA, we therefore draw on a number of psychological treatment strategies to enhance engagement and overcome challenges: psychoeducation, goal setting, self-monitoring of mood and activity, healthy habits, contracting and problem-solving. These strategies are used in a range of psychological therapies and are not specific to Brief BA.

Psychoeducation

'Knowledge is power.' In Brief BA, we aim to work with young people who are struggling with everyday life and often do not know why. We want to build a collaborative and positive therapeutic relationship with them, and help them to take active steps to improve their mood. To do this we try to be as open and transparent as possible. Brief BA has no hidden parts, and everything that happens in treatment should be clear and explicit.

Psychoeducation helps to demystify the experience of depression and its treatment and to develop collaboration between the therapist and young person. Learning that depression is very common can be surprising to a young person and they may find it reassuring to know that their experience is similar to others'. Parents of young people with depression tell us that they often feel powerless to help their son or daughter and do not understand what is happening. As part of Brief BA, we want to give young people and their parents hope that change is possible, and knowledge that they can use. Psychoeducation is therefore a fundamental part of the Brief BA model. We introduce written information leaflets about Brief BA before treatment begins. We then elaborate on this in our first session and provide verbal and written information to take away. We also provide information about where parents and young people can learn more.

Psychoeducation about depression is appreciated by family members (Sanford *et al.* 2006) and improves treatment outcomes for adults with depression, both in terms of how well the person with depression is able to function, and in relation to the wellbeing of their parents or carers (Brady, Kangas and McGill 2017). While there are relatively few studies examining the effect of psychoeducation in the treatment of adolescent depression, Jones *et al.* (2018) reviewed 15 randomized studies. These used a variety of methods including groups, online psychoeducation and individual sessions with parents and young people. The results of this review suggested that psychoeducation has a beneficial effect on a range of measures, including knowledge and understanding of depression and its effects, parent–child communication, treatment adherence and symptoms of depression and other mental health and wellbeing outcomes.

Goal setting

In Brief BA, we want to make a meaningful difference to how young people are able to live and enjoy their life. Young people experience depression in many different ways – Brief BA therefore needs to reflect the individuality of every young person with depression. One way in which we can really reflect each young person is to make sure that we know what they want to achieve. For this reason, when we begin to work with them we need to know what their goals are. We would expect the young person's goals to be linked in some way with the values that they identify in Session 3, 'What matters to you?', and making this link between their treatment goals and their wider values can be very illuminating. If their goals and their values are completely unconnected, it may highlight that either their goals or their values require further discussion and clarification.

Agreement on the goals of therapy is an important part of a positive relationship or alliance between the therapist and the young person (Bordin 1979; Hart 1978). There is extensive and consistent evidence that therapist and client agreement on the goals of therapy is associated with a good treatment outcome (Tryon and Winograd 2002). To be able to agree on the goals of therapy we need to know what the young person's goals are. Interestingly, there is also evidence that identifying positive goals, that is, doing more of something, leads to better outcomes from treatment than goals that are negatively framed, that is, about avoiding something (Wollburg and Braukhaus 2010). This finding fits very well with the approach of Brief BA where we aim to increase valued activities.

In addition to using the individual's personal goals to help build collaboration and a positive therapeutic or working alliance, we can use goals to monitor and track progress in therapy (Weisz *et al.* 2011). We aim to make the treatment goals limited in number and SMART (see Chapter 3) (O'Neill 2000). In Brief BA, we rate the young person's movement towards their goals in every session as part of our Routine Outcome Measures (ROMs) (see Chapter 10). This process is known as goal-based outcomes (GBOs) (Law and Jacob 2015).

Self-monitoring of mood and activity

Early in Brief BA (Session 1), we introduce young people to the idea of recording their daily behaviours and mood. There are a number of very positive reasons for doing this. First is that daily recording of activity (and mood) helps us understand much more quickly the daily life experiences of young people. It helps the therapist and the young person to examine and understand more clearly the link between the young person's behaviour and their mood – and often it will highlight that some activities are associated with more positive moods and that others are associated with more negative mood states. This can help guide the discussion about the young person's values and help choose and structure valued activities.

There is direct evidence that monitoring and tracking our moods and behaviours can improve wellbeing. For example, Burton *et al.* (2013) reviewed the evidence from 16 studies and concluded that simply rating or recording daily activities reduced symptoms of depression and increased wellbeing. Similarly, Kauer *et al.* (2012) found that young people with depression who recorded their activity, mood and stress on their mobile phone significantly reduced their depression symptoms and perceived levels of stress, and became more physically active. Building on this data there are numerous studies demonstrating that if people who are depressed or have symptoms of depression start to become less sedentary, that this leads to reduced depression – this, of course, is the key way that we try to reduce the symptoms of depression in Brief BA.

Although we do not know precisely why recording our moods and activity has a positive impact on wellbeing, there are a number of possible reasons. The first is simply having new information and attending in a more explicit way to our mental state and its fluctuations and changes. This attention also increases our awareness and possibly alters our perspective and ability to self-reflect. This was certainly something that a young woman who had Brief BA told us at the end of treatment:

> '...being able to reflect back on things that we did, made me actively think about it...it kinda kept me thinking about it rather than just allocating this one hour to thinking it through.'

Healthy habits

An important part of Brief BA treatment is identifying the young person's values, that is, 'what matters to you?' We encourage young people to consider different areas of their life and to think about the values that they hold in these different areas. One of the three life areas we focus on is 'me', including the domains of 'physical health' and 'looking after me'. As a result of thinking about their values in relation to themselves, many young people tell us that they want to improve their wellbeing, become more physically fit, and look after their health. Activities and behaviours related to healthy habits are often highly endorsed by parents and they are often able to offer practical support to the young person. However, if you and the young person agree to work on developing healthy habits, it is essential that these are part of the individually tailored content based on a young person's values, in the same way as any other valued activities. As discussed in Part 2, these are strategies young people will often have been 'told' to do by adults (and can often feel patronized or pushed to consider these important), so Brief BA therapists need to make sure they are not repeating unhelpful patterns.

Physical activity

Physical activity can be an important aspect of Brief BA treatment because of the growing evidence that there are consistent and causal relationships between aspects of physical fitness and health, and psychological and mental wellbeing (Schuch *et al.* 2018; Ahn and Fedewa 2011). If young people identify physical fitness as one of their values, we incorporate this into their schedule of valued activities. As always, in scheduling and planning valued activities as part of Brief BA, we encourage young people to break the activity into small steps so that they are more likely to succeed. Depending on the type of physical activity that the young person values, these steps may lead towards solitary, non-competitive and low-impact physical activity, for example walking the dog, walking to college, or at the other extreme, towards more intensive and competitive team sports. It is important to make sure that valued activities reflect the young person's values and not those of their parents, friends or other people.

Two other health-related behaviours that are often mentioned by young people have important associations with depression and low mood, and can be incorporated into valued activities: *sleep* and *diet*.

Sleep

Sleep is one of the most common difficulties that depressed young people report (Goodyer *et al.* 2017), and sleep problems can have a devastating effect on how well they are able to manage in their daily life. Sleep disturbances can exacerbate other depressive symptoms (Spielman and Anderson 1999), and substantially increase the risk of suicidal behaviour and self-harm among depressed adolescents (McCall *et al.* 2010; Singareddy *et al.* 2013). The treatment of choice for sleep difficulties in adults and young people is psychological (Blake *et al.* 2017), and therefore in Brief BA we sometimes use basic psychological techniques to improve sleep, that is, psychoeducation and sleep hygiene. In psychoeducation, we discuss the normal biological changes in sleep and wake cycles that occur during adolescence, and how these conflict with external demands such as having to get up early to attend school. Sleep hygiene steps include simple changes around bedtime routines, lowering their consumption of caffeine, reducing the use of screens (i.e. use of computers and mobile phones) before bedtime, and introducing a regular bedtime and waketime routine (Tan *et al.* 2012). All of these activities can be easily incorporated into the routine scheduling of valued activities.

Diet

There is increasing evidence of a link between depression and our regular diet. This has been reported in adults, where a lifetime-diet rich in fruit and vegetables is associated with a reduced risk of developing depression in later life (Murakami and Sasaki 2010). Similarly, young people who eat unhealthy junk food more frequently tend to report higher symptoms of depression and lower wellbeing than those who eat diets with more vegetables, fruit and complex carbohydrates (Khalid, Williams and Reynolds 2016). There is also evidence that changing diet can improve mood and wellbeing. For example, in a recent randomized controlled trial with 67 adults, Jacka *et al.* (2017) reported that the dietary intervention, promoting a healthy diet with at least nine portions of fruit and vegetables each day, was more effective than social support in reducing symptoms of depression at 12 weeks.

Introducing valued activities related to the young person's diet can be done using standard Brief BA techniques. Young people rarely have full autonomy over their diets, so it may be helpful to involve parents or carers or other family member. Valued activities can include choosing fruit rather than an unhealthy snack, making a healthy packed lunch for school, helping to make a family meal or do the family food shopping, or planning meals for the family. It is important, however, that a parent or carer provides support for the young person and their valued activity, and that any behavioural change is driven by the young person and not by their parent. Diet and nutrition can also be sensitive subjects for some families and can be an area where parents can easily feel blamed by health professionals, so needs to be explored cautiously. In addition, where there are concerns about a young person's weight or eating habits, this is an area of clinical work that should always be discussed in supervision first.

Contracting

Young people (with and without depression) have less autonomy than adults and often do not have access to resources that they need to carry out valued activities. In Brief BA, we want to develop support and structure around young people that will help them increase positive reinforcement and reward and subsequently help them to make the transition from dependence to independence.

Parents and other adults (e.g. teachers, family friends, older siblings, other relatives) are almost always an important part of the emotional and practical support around a young person. However, communication between depressed young people and their potential supporters is often impaired (Sheeber, Hops and Davis 2001). Parent–child interactions are characterized by higher rates of conflict, negative affect and poor problem-solving (Sanders *et al.* 1992) as well as avoidance, which means that the communication between them is ineffective. In this context, it can be difficult for young people to clearly ask for the help that they need, and for parents or other adults to recognize their request and to respond to it. Contracts can be a useful and explicit way of helping the young person access important sources of reward.

The use of family contracts in behavioural therapy appears to have been introduced in the treatment of children and young people with behavioural difficulties (e.g. Stuart 1971). In this context, the primary aim of the contract was to clarify desirable and undesirable behaviours on the part of the child or young person, and the consequences of each (i.e. reinforcement or punishment). Behavioural contracts have also been introduced in family therapy (Falloon 1991) and in marital therapy (Emmelkamp *et al.* 1984).

In Brief BA, we use contracts to help the young person access resources they need to carry out their valued activities. A contract helps them to identify and then ask for, in a very explicit and specific way, the support or help that they need from a parent, carer or other adult. Using a contract can feel artificial, but this can be useful in overcoming some of the common communication patterns that are characteristic of interactions between depressed young people and their parents (e.g. avoidance, conflict). It can reduce any ambiguity and uncertainty about their request. The contract also helps the young person to ask assertively for what they need, to harness the power of the adult's resources and reach a mutual agreement. In Brief BA, the contract is developed between the young person and their adult helper with the support of the therapist.

Problem-solving

Adolescents with depression typically find it difficult to make decisions and have impaired cognitive abilities around organization and planning (see Chapter 9). This difficulty has serious consequences for their functioning and can lead to poor decision-making. There is also evidence that families where there is a young person with depression have more conflict and avoidance and are less efficient at problem-solving than other families with young people who are not depressed (e.g. Sanders *et al.* 1992). For these reasons, we introduce the principles of problem-solving to young people and their parents. In the worksheets, problem-solving is included in Session 6, but it may be used at any point where the young person has a problem to solve.

Problem-solving is a well-established therapeutic technique and is sometimes used as a standalone therapy for adults with depression (e.g. D'Zurilla and Nezu 1986; Nezu, Nezu and Perri 1989). Problem-solving has also been adapted for use with people who have impaired cognitive abilities or problems with impulsivity. For example, Gustavson *et al.* (2016) found that problem-solving was useful when working with older adults with cognitive difficulties. There are a range of studies showing the effects of using problem-solving with young people and their families. For example, family problem-solving was adapted for use with families in which a child or young person had a traumatic brain injury and associated cognitive problems (Wade *et al.* 2018). Family problem-solving improved young people's functioning at school and work and was particularly helpful for young people who had parents with fewer years of formal education. Problem-solving can also be useful for adolescents who have autistic spectrum disorders (ASD) and struggle in social situations (Bonete, Calero and Fernández-Parra 2015), and with young people who have behavioural as well as emotional difficulties (Sanders *et al.* 1992).

The technique of problem-solving offers a flexible, clear, generalizable and structured, step-by-step approach. It can be particularly useful in helping young people and parents overcome misunderstanding and disagreements. Parents have often used the technique of problem-solving in their work or home life, and therefore find it familiar and credible. Problem-solving starts by describing and defining the problem that is being addressed. This can help clarify differences between the young person and the parent's or carer's perspectives. Generating possible solutions means that people have to take a step back and take a more creative and open-minded approach. It also means that parents and young people start to share responsibility for solving the problem, and this can influence family interactions.

CHAPTER 14

The Evidence Base for Behavioural Activation for Depression

The aim of Brief BA is to offer treatment that helps young people recover from depression and get back to their normal lives as soon as possible. There are a number of different types of BA, ranging in length and complexity. In this chapter, we will review the evidence for the effectiveness of BA, in general and in relation to young people with depression. To help put this into context we will also briefly describe other evidence-based treatments for depression and the method used to evaluate if a treatment is effective or not effective.

Types of Behavioural Activation therapy

The behavioural treatment of depression is based on a well-established theory (Lewinsohn 1974). Currently there are three main types of BA that vary mainly in their complexity and length:

- Christopher Martell and colleagues (Martell, Addis and Jacobson 2001) developed the most complex version of BA for depression, which aims to do three main things: (i) increase engagement in adaptive activities (which are often those associated with the experience of pleasure or mastery); (ii) decrease engagement in activities that maintain depression or increase risk for depression; and (iii) solve problems that limit access to reward or that maintain or increase aversive control. This version of BA incorporates a detailed analysis of behaviour to identify personal reinforcers, and also includes techniques to address the problem of rumination (repetitive, negative thinking). Treatment typically lasts for between 16 and 20 weeks.
- *BA for the treatment of depression (BATD)* was developed as a more concise version by Lejuez, Hopko and Hopko (2001) and Lejuez *et al.* (2011). To combat problems associated with shortages of qualified therapists and low funding levels, BATD was designed to be simple and able to be delivered in five to ten sessions by a therapist who did not have formal training in psychotherapy. Brief BA, as described in this manual, was designed from BATD.
- *Activity scheduling* (Cuijpers, van Straten and Warmerdam 2007) is routinely used in low-intensity psychological therapy services for adults as well as many other settings. It is delivered by Psychological Wellbeing Practitioners and clinicians with one year of clinical training but who do not have training in a formal psychotherapy. The aim is usually to increase routine,

necessary and pleasurable activities, although variations on the type of activities are found in different versions.

Evidence-based psychological therapies for young people with depression

A range of evidence-based psychological therapies for adolescents with depression is available. These have all been shown to be effective at reducing the symptoms of depression in young people (NICE 2019), and may be available in routine mental health services.

Cognitive behaviour therapy (CBT)

Cognitive behaviour therapy (CBT) for depression is based on the idea that depression is linked to, and maintained by, a range of cognitions (thoughts) and behaviours. People with depression also hold a range of negative thoughts about themselves (e.g. 'I'm useless'), the world (e.g. 'Everything is awful') and the future (e.g. 'Nothing will ever get better'). These negative thoughts appear to be true and believable and make people feel even worse. CBT aims to treat depression by helping individuals to identify and then challenge their negative thoughts, and to identify links between their behaviours and their moods and then increase behaviours that improve mood and reduce behaviours that make them feel worse (IMPACT 2010). The behavioural part of CBT is very similar to BA, and the early evidence for BA came from a study that aimed to 'dismantle' CBT and identify the most effective part.

Interpersonal therapy (IPT)

Interpersonal therapy (IPT) focuses on the way in which personal roles and relationships with other people are related to depression (Mufson *et al.* 2015). In therapy, the client and therapist identify changes in key areas of life that may be associated with or have triggered depression. These are varied and may include changes in school or work, family changes, such as parental divorce or separation, bereavement, or loss of important personal relationships, for example breaking up with a girlfriend or boyfriend. IPT also considers conflict with others or isolation and loneliness as possible areas of interest. The focus of therapy is on building interpersonal skills to overcome relationship difficulties, problem-solving difficulties and improving communication with others. Parents may be invited to join therapy sessions if family conflict or changes in family relationships are identified as important.

Systemic family therapy (SFT)

Systemic approaches to therapy for depression view the problems experienced by one individual as reflecting wider issues in the family 'system' (Cottrell and Boston 2002). In a system, changes in any one element (a family member) impact on and reverberate around the system and affect everyone. Systemic family therapy (SFT) therefore treats a depressed adolescent in the context of their wider family and possibly even wider systems, including the school and peer group. Usually, other family members are invited into sessions and help to identify the potential causes of depression in the young person as well as working out how to bring about change.

Identifying evidence-based treatments – the randomized controlled trial (RCT)

The best way to test the effectiveness of a treatment is to compare it to another treatment. Any new treatment should be at least as good as an existing treatment. Ideally, the new treatment will also be cheaper or no more expensive than the existing treatment, and will have no extra side effects or complications. The best kind of study to test if a new treatment is effective is a randomized controlled trial (RCT).

The RCT is a special kind of comparative study used to evaluate healthcare treatments. In an RCT, two or more treatments are compared in as fair a way as is possible. Usually, a new treatment is compared to an existing treatment. There are clear rules and regulations about how to run an RCT and researchers are expected to follow these and to share their data so that other researchers can check their findings. The rules of the RCT are there to make sure that people who help with an RCT are treated with respect, compassion and fairness, to be as sure as possible that the comparison is fair and that the data collected is accurate and analysed correctly.

RCT 'rules' are as follows:

- Everyone who takes part in the study (known as a 'participant') is given clear information about the study, what will be involved, and if there are any risks of taking part
- Everyone who takes part in the study must give fully informed consent – this means that they understand what the study is about and are happy to take part. If the person is under 16 years old their parent has to give consent and the young person also has to agree to take part – this is called 'assent'
- Participants can leave the study at any time without having to give a reason
- Participants are *randomized* to the different treatments. This means that everyone gets the same chance to be offered the new treatment or the existing treatment, and there is no way of predicting or influencing who gets what treatment. Ideally, the randomization is done completely independently of the research team
- Ideally, participants and researchers do not know if they are getting the new treatment or the existing treatment. This is known as *double blinding*, that is, both the participant and the researchers are *blind* to what treatment group they are in. Blinding is usual in RCTs of new drugs because drugs can be made to look the same. Blinding is not usually possible in psychological therapy trials because participants (and therapists) know what form of psychological therapy they are receiving. So, in a psychological therapy RCT, only the researchers are blind to the treatment allocation – the study is *single blind*
- Before the study begins the researchers nominate the most important way that they will measure improvement or change in symptoms and when they will measure it. So, in a study about the treatment of depression, the researchers decide what measure of depression is *primary* and when they will measure it. This is usually the participant's own report about their symptoms – but it could also be a report by a carer or parent, or by a clinician – or a change in behaviour. The measure is taken at the end of treatment and later, after treatment ends. One time point and one measure combine to the *primary outcome measure*. Having a clear primary outcome measure means that researchers cannot choose the best measure that suits their purpose or hypothesis or choose when they compare the new and existing treatments

- Researchers must also monitor, record and report bad things that happen to participants. This is so that 'adverse' events can be measured and any risks associated with the new or existing treatments picked up and compared
- All the participants who get randomized are monitored and accounted for at the end of the study – even if they drop out of treatment. This is to make sure that the results are not distorted by having more people drop out of one treatment than another, and then only collecting the primary outcome measure from those who stay in the treatments to the end
- There is an independent statistician to calculate the effects of the new and existing treatments, to make sure that the results are treated fairly and that no bias can be introduced (either by accident or intentionally).

RCTs take a long time to run, involve a lot of participants, and usually a large research team with different kinds of experts, including people who have had the condition (in this case, depression), and can represent the views of other patients and often their carers. Larger RCTs with more participants give results that are more reliable. However, RCTs are expensive. Sometimes because of the costs involved they are not large enough to give a reliable result. This can lead to a lot of smaller studies and no one study that is really large enough to be conclusive. To overcome this problem there is a way of combining the results of many different studies and data from all the people who took part in them so that there can be a stronger test of the new treatment. This combination of treatment studies is called a meta-analysis.

How well does BA work?

The first RCT to examine the efficacy of BA as a treatment for depression was conducted by Neil Jacobson and colleagues (1996). Their aim was to compare two active components of CBT – behavioural activation (B) and cognitive restructuring (C). People who had depression were therefore randomized to receive full CBT, or cognitive restructuring, or behavioural activation. To the researchers' surprise (and contrary to their hypotheses) behavioural activation was just as effective as cognitive restructuring and was as effective as the full conventional CBT treatment.

Once the initial study had shown that BA was effective in treating depression, it was tested in a range of different studies with adults attending mental health outpatient services as well as with many other different types of people. These include:

- Older adults (Pasterfield *et al.* 2014)
- New mothers (O'Mahen *et al.* 2013)
- People with learning difficulties (Jahoda *et al.* 2017)
- People with chronic pain (Hooker *et al.* 2019)
- Women with breast cancer (Ryba, Lejuez, and Hopko 2014).

BA has also been delivered in different ways – this is usually to try to make it easier and less expensive and also easier for people who have depression to access it. Dave Richards and colleagues (2016) conducted a large study in the UK. Their aim was to assess if BA was as effective and cost-effective as CBT in the treatment of depression. Four hundred and forty adults with depression were randomized to receive BA, which was delivered by Psychological Wellbeing Practitioners, therapists who have one year of training and no training in formal psychological therapy, or CBT, which was delivered by accredited and fully trained CBT therapists.

The results of the study showed that CBT was no more effective than BA in treating depression. Importantly, BA was more cost-effective than CBT because the costs of delivering BA treatment were less than the costs of CBT. This is important because it means that, given the same budget, more people can be treated with BA than with CBT.

Enthusiasm for BA has also led to developments in how it is delivered. BA has been delivered to groups of patients as well as to individuals (Porter, Spates and Smitham 2004) and online (Puspitasari *et al.* 2013). BA has also been delivered by a range of people, including those with minimal clinical experience and training (e.g. Acierno *et al.* 2016). To test if these various versions of BA are effective and safe, Dave Ekers and colleagues (2011, 2014) have reviewed and integrated the research data from all available studies. Their results show that BA is effective when used with many different groups of people. Importantly, simple and brief BA was just as effective as more complicated and longer BA. This is important because if treatment is simple, it can be delivered by more people, and if treatment is brief, more people can be treated in the same period of time.

So, with adults:

- BA is at least as effective as other evidence-based treatments for depression
- BA is less costly than other evidence-based treatments for depression
- BA can be delivered in a range of different ways
- Simple and brief BA is as effective as more complex and longer BA.

Does BA work with depressed adolescents?

The characteristics of BA – relatively simple, brief and effective – mean that it is a plausible and attractive treatment for adolescent depression. Surprisingly, however, given the challenges of treating young people who have depression, there has not been much research on the effectiveness of BA with young people. Fortunately, the work that has been done suggests that BA is both effective and safe when used to treat depression in this population. Most of this research consists of individual case reports, where researchers have evaluated BA with one or two young people. There is also one case series, which includes 20 young people and two small RCTs.

McCauley *et al.* (2016) assessed if BA is effective for adolescents with depression. This study was carried out in the USA. Sixty depressed young people aged 12 to 18 were recruited and randomized to receive either BA or another evidence-based therapy (either IPT or CBT). BA was based on the Martell model, adapted for adolescents, and included 14 sessions of treatment delivered over 12 weeks. Symptoms of depression were assessed at the start and end of therapy and six months and one year after therapy began. At the end of treatment young people in both treatment groups reported statistically significant reductions in depression symptoms, and there were no differences between the two groups. Also in the USA, Chu and colleagues (2016) evaluated group BA for adolescents with anxiety and depression in a small randomized trial with 35 young people who were randomized to receive BA or were kept on a waiting list. At the end of BA treatment the young people reported significant reductions in depression and anxiety and symptoms were significantly lower in the BA group compared to the waiting list control group. The effectiveness of BA for adolescent depression has been integrated and reviewed in two separate studies (Martin and Oliver 2018; Tindall *et al.* 2017). Both reviews acknowledged the scarcity of high-quality research but found that the preliminary evidence supported that effectiveness of BA for young people.

These promising studies from the USA encouraged us to adapt BA for depressed adolescents who were being treated in Child and Adolescent Mental Health services in the UK. In this context, where services are publicly funded and free at the point of delivery, it is very important to introduce treatments that are flexible and cost-effective. In addition, because highly qualified therapists are scarce, and because Ekers *et al.* (2014) found no difference in effectiveness between complex and more simple BA, we decided to adapt the brief form of BA, BATD (Lejuez *et al.* 2011).

With the help of the originator of BATD, Carl Lejuez, young people, their parents and trainee therapists, we developed Brief BA, specifically for young people with depression. When we develop or adapt a treatment it is important to check that it is safe and effective. This is usually done in a couple of small studies where careful attention can be given to individual patients, and where any safety issues can be quickly spotted (see the references listed below).

PUBLICATIONS DESCRIBING THE USE AND OUTCOMES OF BRIEF BA IN THE UK

Pass, L., Lejuez, C.W. and Reynolds, S. (2018) 'Brief behavioural activation (Brief BA) for adolescent depression: A pilot study.' *Behavioural and Cognitive Psychotherapy 46*(2), 182–194. [A report of the first 20 young people who received Brief BA for depression. It describes the key treatment outcomes.]

Pass, L., Whitney, H. and Reynolds, S. (2016) 'Brief behavioral activation for adolescent depression: Working with complexity and risk.' *Clinical Case Studies 15*(5), 360–375. [Describes the use of Brief BA with a young person who had reported suicidal thoughts.]

Pass, L., Hodgson, E., Whitney, H. and Reynolds, S. (2018) 'Brief behavioral activation treatment for depressed adolescents delivered by nonspecialist clinicians: A case illustration.' *Cognitive and Behavioral Practice 25*(2), 208–224. [Outlines the delivery of Brief BA by a trainee therapist who had no formal training in psychological therapy.]

Pass, L., Sancho, M., Brett, S., Jones, M. and Reynolds, S. (2018) 'Brief Behavioural Activation (Brief BA) in secondary schools: A feasibility study examining acceptability and practical considerations.' *Educational and Child Psychology 35*(2). [Describes the delivery of Brief BA in secondary schools, and considers how it might need to be adapted.]

Each of these articles uses data from the Routine Outcome Measures (ROMs) that are incorporated into the treatment. Therefore, the Brief BA approach includes simple measures of symptoms, functioning and wellbeing (ROMs) that young people complete and share with their therapist at every session. This means that the therapist and young person can see if things are getting better or worse, and focus the treatment accordingly. The session-by-session measures also show how symptoms and functioning change from the beginning to the end of treatment, and can then be used to evaluate the effectiveness of treatment. This is always important, but especially so when there is limited data from RCTs that we can use.

In the case series (Pass, Lejeuz and Reynolds, 2018), 20 young people who had been referred to the NHS and been given a diagnosis of depression were offered Brief BA. Treatment was delivered by a range of different professionals, including a psychology assistant, Psychological Wellbeing Practitioner and a postgraduate student. All were supervised by a clinical psychologist. At the end of treatment the young people's symptoms were significantly reduced. Very encouragingly, only one young person did not complete treatment – suggesting that the treatment was acceptable and engaging to young people. Most young people in the study were discharged at the end of Brief BA treatment; some were referred onwards for other difficulties, including an eating disorder, anxiety and family problems. No young person required additional psychological therapy for depression.

Currently, therefore, we have been encouraged that the available evidence suggests that BA is likely to be as effective and safe as existing evidence-based psychological therapy in treating young people who have depression. However, we are also cautious and are acutely aware that the evidence is limited. There is no RCT that has been conducted in the UK or in any publicly funded health service. The only RCT using a contemporary individual BA approach is small and was carried out in a university clinic in the USA rather than in routine clinical practice. Data from our clinic in the UK does not include an RCT, but the participants were referred and treated in a UK mental health service, and are therefore likely to be broadly similar to other depressed young people referred to NHS services.

There is obviously an urgent need for a large, well-designed RCT to be conducted in the UK to assess if Brief BA is effective, cost-effective and safe when used to treat adolescents with depression. There is increasing demand for treatment for adolescents with depression and too few qualified therapists to meet the demand. Existing evidence-based therapies all require lengthy periods of training, and there is currently no well-established evidence-based low-intensity treatment for adolescents with depression. Until we are able to base clinical practice on well-designed RCTs, it will be essential to keep the safety and effectiveness of Brief BA under review, using ROMs, completed by young people, to assess improvement and deterioration of symptoms, functioning and risk.

PART 4

BRIEF BA SESSION CHECKLISTS AND WORKSHEETS

Contents

All pages marked ✦ in Part 4 can be photocopied and downloaded at https://library.jkp.com/redeem using the code TAUPAGE for personal use with this programme.

Brief BA Assessment Checklist

Brief BA Assessment Checklist *Please note that this will also need to cover all your specific service requirements*	
Complete?	**Task**
	Introductions (introduce self, ask young person preferred name, outline assessment process and length, agree how to split time with young person and parent and young person alone)
	Explain audio/video recording and complete consent form(s) as applicable
	Turn audio/video recorder on
	Explain confidentiality, limits to this (if risk of harm to young person or others)
	Anything in particular to make time for today? Details:
	Explain use of ROMs and how they inform assessment and treatment planning
	Young person symptom questionnaire (e.g. full RCADS)
	Young person functioning/quality of life questionnaire (e.g. ORS)
	Parent report of young person symptom questionnaire (e.g. full RCADS-P)
	Parent report of young person functioning/quality of life questionnaire (e.g. ORS)
	Assess depression symptoms: • Anhedonia • Irritability and depressed mood • Suicidal thoughts • Sleep problems • Fatigue • Cognitive problems • Appetite or weight change • Negative self-perceptions • Psychomotor changes
	Comprehensive risk assessment (suicidal thoughts, plans or actions, self-harm, other risks to self, risk to others, risk from others)
	Create safety plan
	Other service-specific assessment actions:
	Identify possible goals for therapy and rate them on 0–10 scale
	Photocopy completed young person session worksheet
	Give 'An Information Leaflet for Young People' (if appropriate at this stage)
	Give 'An Information Leaflet for Parents, Carers and Other Adults' (if appropriate at this stage)
	Confirm next steps (what happens next, when, where, who with)
	Young person session feedback questionnaire (e.g. SRS)
	Parent session feedback questionnaire (e.g. SRS)

After assessment	
Complete?	**Task**
	Upload audio/video recording and delete from device
	Score young person + parent ROMs (if not done in session)
	Complete any electronic/paper client record keeping actions required
	Electronic or paper session record: ROMs, risk, attendees, content, next steps or appointment
	Upload completed session worksheets and ROMs to electronic records (if applicable)
	Diary appointment for next session
	Prepare to discuss in supervision and/or wider team meeting for treatment planning
	Book room for next session

Safety Plan

Many young people can have times where things feel overwhelming and they can't cope. This is a practical plan with some coping strategies to use if you are distressed, and to help you stay safe.

My warning signs/triggers that I can identify early:

....

....

Things that have helped in the past that might work now:

....

....

Other ways I can look after myself:

....

....

New strategies I can try (e.g. letting someone know, staying in a public area, doing something to distract me):

....

....

What things help lift my mood?

....

....

What things are good at distracting me from these kinds of thoughts?

....

....

What would I say to someone close to me who was feeling this way?

....

....

Help from others

Relative:

....

Friend:

....

Professional:

....

To stay safe, I can call:

....

Somewhere safe I can go:

....

Brief BA: Pre-Session 1 Checklist

ID/Client initials:

Date:

Complete?	Task
	Read all available: • Electronic or paper notes • Letters • Reports
	Discuss with supervisor: • Who to invite to Session 1 • Any key issues to consider? • Confirm availability of senior staff for risk discussion
	Post out or send: • Appointment confirmation • 'An Information Leaflet for Young People' • 'An Information Leaflet for Parents, Carers and Other Adults' • Any directions or parking information
	Prepare Session 1 materials: • Session checklist • Audio/video recorder (check batteries, memory, cables required) • Consent forms (as applicable for service, team, role) • Young person Session 1 worksheets • Parent Session 1 worksheets • Young person Session 1 ROMs • Parent Session 1 ROMs
	Other service-specific preparation tasks (e.g. lone working requirements, car pool booking, video recorder loan request): __________ __________ __________
	Book room
	Add diary appointment to electronic or paper record system

An Information Leaflet for Young People

What is depression?

Depression includes a combination of difficulties including low mood, irritability and not enjoying life. Problems with sleep, eating and activity are very common, and young people can feel worthless and sometimes see no point in living. Depression is more common than you might think and can affect any of us. It can be a result of many different things. Often depression is triggered by a bad experience, a loss or failure, or a combination of bad experiences. Low mood and other symptoms of depression impact on how we think, feel and behave, and interfere with our everyday life.

This is a vicious cycle of depression that people can often find themselves stuck in. They feel depressed, so they do less of what matters to them, but because of this they get less of the 'feel-good factor' from life, and so feel even worse.

'Doing more of what matters' can have an enormous impact on our mood by:

- Making us feel better about ourselves
- Making us feel less tired
- Increasing motivation
- Giving us a sense of achievement.

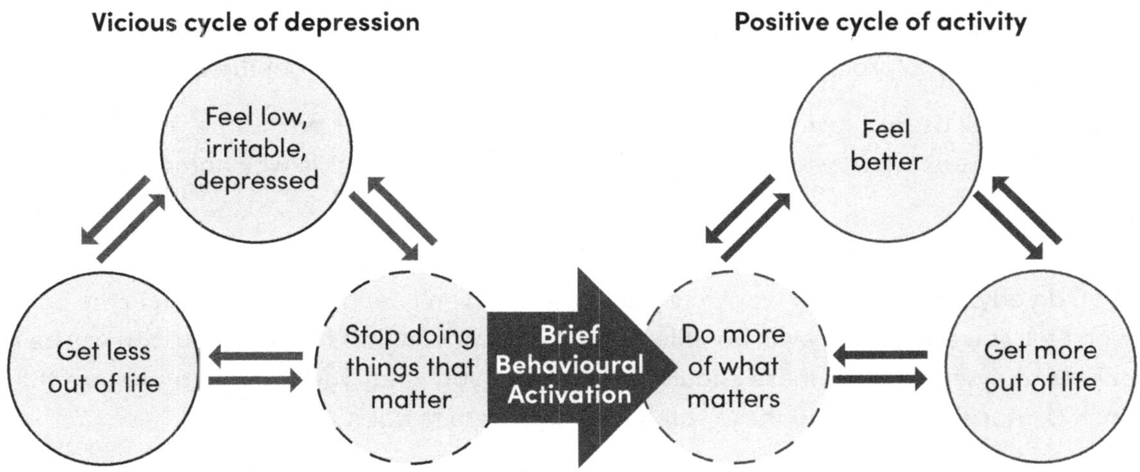

THE BRIEF BA MODEL

How can Brief Behavioural Activation (Brief BA) help me?

Brief Behavioural Activation (Brief BA) is a talking therapy for depression. It is also a 'doing therapy'. It is based on the idea that by doing more valued activities, people will start to feel better. Sounds too simple, right? Well, actually it's not as simple as it sounds, and that's why we work together to make it fit for you. Research into BA suggests it is an effective way of treating depression by breaking the vicious cycle pictured.

In Brief BA, we will help you to do more of what matters to *you*. When you start to do more of what matters to you, you will start to get more out of life – more of the feel-good factor. When you get more out of life you start to feel slightly better. Feeling slightly better will make it easier to do a bit more of what matters...so you will get more out of life and feel a bit better. It's a positive cycle now.

We will help you select different activities across different areas of your life. We will help you find activities that fall into one of the categories below:

Achievement	**Closeness**	**Enjoyable**	**Important**
Did you get something out of the activity? Were you pleased when it was done and out of the way?	Did the activity made you feel close to anyone, even if you weren't with them?	Did you enjoy the activity? Was it fun?	Was the activity important to *you*?

For example, if you went to play football you might find that this ticks all of those boxes. Doing work for school or college may be important, but not enjoyable. However, it still has to be done – and doesn't it feel good when you do hand in that piece of homework? So you would also get something in the Achievement box.

The idea with Brief BA is that if you can get a *balance* of valued activities each week then you will start to feel better, as you are doing things that matter to you and so getting more out of life.

How does Brief BA work?

Your therapist will support you using Brief BA. They will be like a coach, teaching you the skills for Brief BA, but you will need to go away and give it a go. Like if you were learning to play the guitar, your music teacher will teach you how to play certain notes but you would need to go away and practise. The more you practise the easier it will become, and you will get the most out of Brief BA.

The treatment will usually last for eight sessions, for about an hour each time. That means there are 167 hours a week when you are not with your therapist, and this is why home activities are so important!

In each session, you and your therapist will pick the tasks together for the next week. They won't ever make you do anything you don't want to do, and if you haven't been able to complete the activities, they won't tell you off! But they will be able to help you work on that for next time. You will be given worksheets at every session; these should help remind you what you need to do before the next session. It is important you keep these safe and bring them to each session.

Every week your Brief BA therapist will ask you to complete some brief questionnaires about how things are going for you, so you can track your progress through sessions and identify any particular problems, set-backs or symptoms that might be getting in the way. They will also ask you to give feedback on the session each time, so they can make Brief BA work best for *you*.

Getting parents involved...

All sessions will take place with you, but there will be times we'll ask your parents or guardians to join us to keep them updated on how you are doing, to discuss tasks that you are setting over the next week, or because we may need their help in some way. It can also be a good idea to share your tasks with your parents or guardians so they know what you have planned over the week, and can give you help if you need it.

Things feeling really difficult?

A common symptom of depression is having thoughts of 'not wanting to be here anymore' or of hurting yourself in some way. Throughout treatment your therapist needs to make sure that you can keep yourself safe, and will ask you questions about this. So if you are having these thoughts, speak to your therapist about them, or if you need to speak to someone straightaway, see the contact box below.

You can also use your safety plan to help when you're feeling really low – we'll complete this at your first session.

Remember, it is important to tell someone about these thoughts if you are experiencing them. They are a normal symptom of depression, but you don't have to listen to them.

Any questions? Please ask – we're happy to discuss anything you want to know.

If you need help right now you can contact: Contact name: Tel: Non-urgent contact details:

An Information Leaflet for Parents, Carers and Other Adults

What is depression?

Depression includes a combination of difficulties including low mood, irritability and not enjoying life. Problems with sleep, eating, thinking and activity are very common, and young people often feel worthless and see no point in living. It is common for young people with depression to isolate themselves, to feel self-critical, and lack energy. Up to one in four young people will experience an episode of depression by the time they turn 18.

Depression can affect any of us. It can be a result of many different things. Often depression is triggered by a bad experience, a loss or failure, or a combination of bad experiences. Sometimes it can be hard to identify any particular trigger. Symptoms of depression impact on how we think, feel and behave, and interfere with our everyday life.

This is the vicious cycle of depression that people can often find themselves stuck in. When we feel depressed, we often do less of what matters to us, but because of this we can get less of the 'feel-good factor' from life, and so feel even worse. By increasing meaningful activity we can see a big improvement in mood levels.

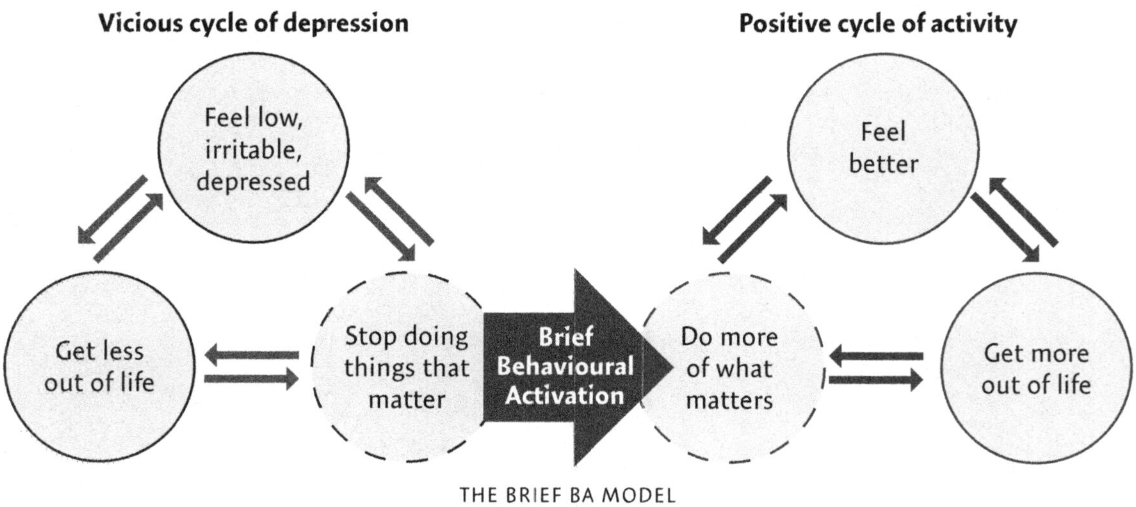

THE BRIEF BA MODEL

How can Brief Behavioural Activation (Brief BA) help my child?

Brief BA is used to treat depression. It is based on the idea that by doing more activities that are personally important, people start to feel better. There has been a lot of research into BA, which has found that it is an effective way of treating depression by breaking the vicious cycle and creating a positive cycle.

Brief BA is not just encouraging your child to do more activities – they might be doing lots already. The idea of Brief BA is encouraging a balance of meaningful, valued activities for your son or daughter based on what *they* find important.

For example, someone may spend their days either at school, doing homework in the evening, or talking to school friends on social media. This means that everything they do is linked to school in some way. Could you imagine if something went wrong at school? The smallest problem could become a disaster when there isn't a healthy balance. The aim of Brief BA is to increase the range of different activities that your son or daughter is doing that they find important and rewarding, and to get these rewards from different areas of life.

In Brief BA, the young person will be encouraged to record their activities outside sessions, as well as complete some brief questionnaires each time they meet the therapist to check on how they are doing. Recording activities is important, as the therapist will use the records during each session to monitor progress and troubleshoot any issues.

The therapist will also help your son or daughter identify and schedule a balance of activities that fall into one of the categories below:

Achievement	**Closeness**	**Enjoyable**	**Important**
Did your child get anything out of the activity? Were they glad when it was done?	Did the activity make your child feel close to anyone?	Did your child enjoy the activity?	Was the activity important to your child?

How many sessions will there be?

There are usually eight sessions, plus a review around a month after Session 8. We try to have two sessions a week at first to get going quickly. Each session will last for about an hour. Most of the sessions will just be the young person and the therapist. However, in Sessions 1, 6 and 8, we will invite you and/or other important adults to join us. We may also contact you between sessions to give you an update.

How do the sessions work?

Brief BA is a very practical therapy so it will require a little effort from the young person in between sessions. It is like learning any new skill - the more you practise, the better you will become. In each session, the young person and the therapist will pick tasks together for the young person to do over the next week. Then, in the next session, they will review how they went. If there are any problems with the tasks, that's fine - the therapist will be able to help work on that for next time.

The young person will be given worksheets that will be partly filled out in session and partly at home. This will remind them of what they need to do in between sessions. It is important that these are brought to each session, as reviewing these will form part of the session. You will also be given your own worksheets that explain what is being covered in each Brief BA session, and how you can support this work at home.

What can I do?

You can help your son or daughter by being as positive as you can and giving them praise and encouragement for every effort they make, no matter how small. Getting over depression is hard.

Brief BA involves acting 'from the outside in'. Rather than waiting until they feel better and then doing things, your child will be asked to do valued activities even when they feel low or bad or unmotivated. The idea is that this valued activity creates reward, or the 'feel-good factor'. There will probably be times when your son or daughter doesn't want to do the activity because they feel too tired or 'don't see the point'. This is where you can help and support. It will be important to encourage them to stick to the plan and try the activity anyway. You can remind them that the process takes time and that people don't feel better overnight. You can also help them by talking about what might make it easier for them to do these activities, such as someone else doing it with them, or getting help with the first few steps.

What if my child is really struggling?

A common symptom of depression is having thoughts of 'not wanting to be here anymore' or of hurting yourself in some way. Your son or daughter may report having these thoughts at some point. It is important that the therapist is aware of these thoughts as they need to make sure that the young person can keep themselves safe throughout treatment. You may be included in a safety plan that is agreed with your child. If your child is struggling with these thoughts, you can use these contact numbers shown below for support. Your child can also make use of these numbers themselves. Talking about these kinds of thoughts does not make it more likely that someone will act on them, so don't be afraid to speak with your child and let them know you are there to help.

Any questions? Please ask – we're happy to discuss any questions or concerns you may have.

Non-urgent contact:
Email:
Tel:
Emergency contact:
Tel:

Brief BA Session 1 Checklist

ID/Client initials:

Date:

Brief BA Session 1 Checklist	
Complete?	**Task**
	Introductions (introduce self, ask young person preferred name, outline session and length, agree how to split time with young person and parent but also with young person alone)
	Explain audio/video recording and complete consent form(s) as applicable
	Turn audio/video recorder on
	Explain confidentiality, limits to this (if risk of harm to young person or others)
	Anything in particular to make time for today? Details:
	Explain use of ROMs and how they inform therapy
	Complete ROMs: • Young person symptom questionnaire (e.g. RCADS Depression Subscale + Risk Q, or full RCADS if not done recently) • Young person functioning/quality of life questionnaire (e.g. ORS) • Parent report of young person symptom questionnaire (e.g. RCADS Depression Subscale + Risk Q, or full RCADS if not done recently) • Parent report of young person functioning/quality of life questionnaire (e.g. ORS)
	Risk discussion and check on changes since assessment
	Safety plan review
	Introduce Brief BA
	Overview of depression: explore current symptoms
	Ask about possible triggers
	Explain Brief BA maintenance cycle
	Set goals and rate them on 0–10 scale (or if already completed, review and rate)
	Introduce activity log
	Fill in activity log for day before
	Agree homework: complete activity log, read worksheets
	Photocopy completed young person's session worksheets
	Give young person session worksheets to take away
	Give parent session worksheets to take away
	Confirm next session date, time, location
	Young person session feedback questionnaire (e.g. SRS)
	Parent session feedback questionnaire (e.g. SRS)

After Session 1	
Complete?	**Task**
	Upload audio/video recording and delete from device
	Score young person and parent ROMs (if not done in session)
	Outcome electronic diary appointment (if applicable)
	Electronic or paper session record: ROMs, risk, attendees, content, homework, next appointment
	Upload completed session worksheets and ROMs to electronic records (if applicable)
	Diary appointment for next session
	Prepare to discuss in supervision
	Book room for next session

Young Person Brief BA Session 1 Worksheet

[Therapist photo here]

Introductions

Therapist's name: **[Full name]**

Contact number: **[Service contact number]**

About depression

Depression is a problem that many teenagers face, and affects how we feel, our thoughts, our behaviours and our bodies. For some it comes out of the blue, while others have been trying to cope with it for a long time.

Up to 25% of young people will have experienced depression by the time they are 18.

When you are depressed, you may notice a number of changes. Those listed below are common and you may have others that are not listed here. Do you recognize many?

- Losing interest or enjoyment, finding things are no longer fun
- Feeling depressed, down, sad or irritable
- Increase or decrease in appetite or weight
- Thinking about death and dying, suicide
- Extreme tiredness, fatigue
- Sleeping too much or not enough
- Difficulties concentrating or making decisions
- Feeling worthless or guilty
- Not wanting to be around people
- Physical agitation or slowness

My other depression symptoms:

What causes depression?

It is difficult to say why someone gets depressed as everybody is different, and there is no one specific cause for depression. Sometimes the reason may be obvious; sometimes it might not be clear.

Jayden is 17 years old and started feeling low when he started struggling with his IT course at college; he recently dropped out after missing a load of teaching and found it really hard to catch up. He has a Saturday job but hasn't gone recently. His friends are busy with work or college, and his dad struggles with his own depression at times so he doesn't want to bother him. He feels down and irritable most of the time, and often snaps at people for no reason. Jayden sleeps a lot during the day as well as at night. His family have noticed that he seems slowed down. Jayden has stopped seeing his friends as he can't be bothered to go out and everything seems like a huge effort. He hates himself and at times has wished he wasn't here.

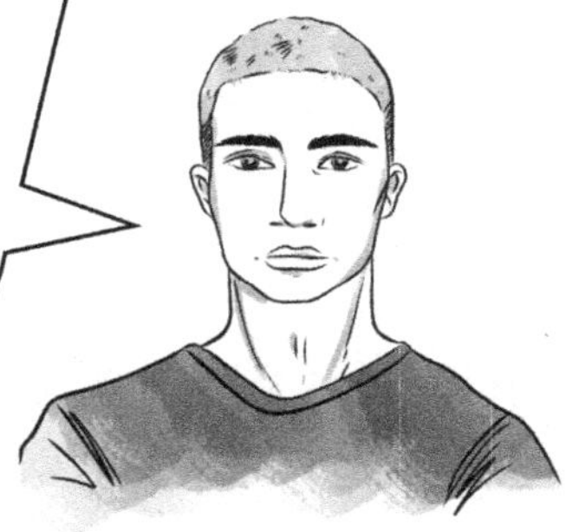

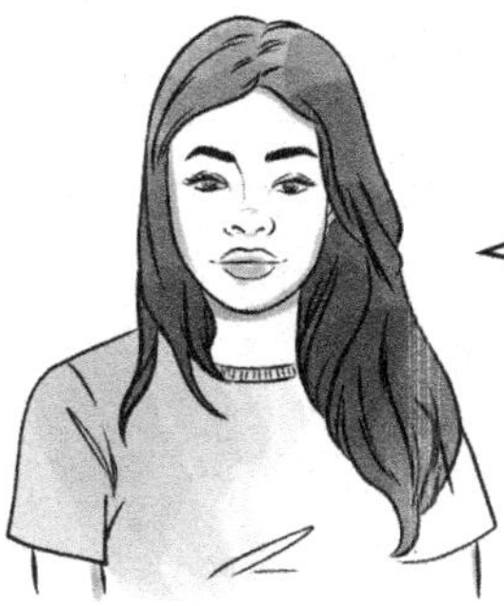

Sofia is 16 years old. Her low mood started after her gran died last year, and things gradually got worse. Also, her best friend has recently got a new girlfriend, meaning he doesn't see as much of Sofia. Sofia feels down most days, cries a lot of the time and finds it a real struggle to concentrate on homework. Even though she still goes to school and has dance classes twice a week, she feels as if she isn't enjoying anything she does. Sofia finds it hard to get to sleep, and often wakes up in the middle of the night. She has lost her appetite since she started feeling low, and only eats when her mum makes her. She thinks she is a failure and that things are never going to improve.

Possible triggers for my depression:

The here and now

Don't worry if you're not sure what might have triggered your depression in the first place. The important thing for us to think about together is what's happening now, and what can be changed to help you feel better. Depression can be a 'vicious cycle', where the more depressed you feel, the less you want to do, and the less you do (especially less of the things that matter), the less you get out of life and the more depressed you feel.

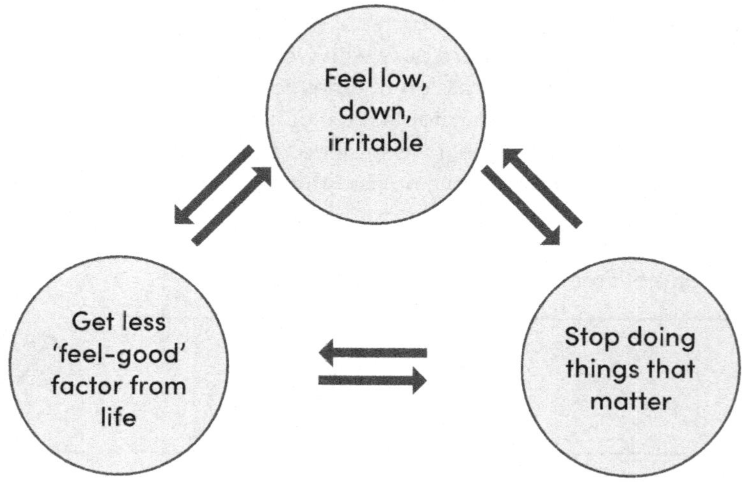

THE VICIOUS CYCLE OF DEPRESSION

The key to feeling better is in understanding what is keeping depression going. Doing things differently can help you think and feel differently.

The Brief Behavioural Activation (Brief BA) approach

Brief Behavioural Activation (Brief BA) is based on the idea that your ability to feel better has a lot to do with how you live your life on a day-to-day basis.

This treatment focuses on helping you develop different patterns of behaviour where you do valued activities every day that help you break out of this vicious cycle and start to feel better.

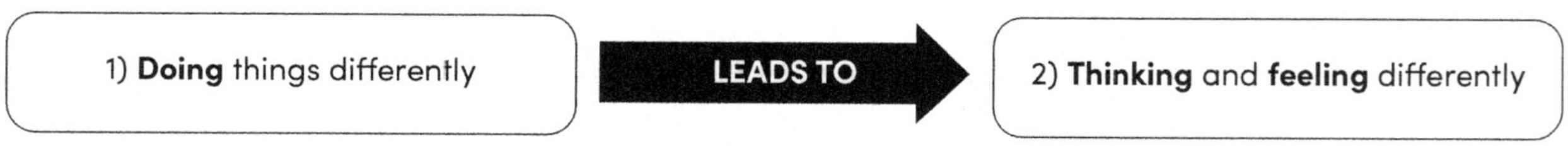

1) **Doing** things differently
LEADS TO
2) **Thinking** and **feeling** differently

BEATING DEPRESSION WITH BRIEF BEHAVIOURAL ACTIVATION

Lots of research has shown that BA is an effective way of treating low mood in both adults and young people.

Brief BA is all about *increasing* activities that are helpful and important to you, and *reducing* unhelpful activities.

Introducing the activity log

Because the main focus of Brief BA is increasing healthy (non-depressed) behaviour, it's important for us to get a sense of exactly how you are spending each day. You probably feel you already have a good sense of how you spend your time, but the purpose of the activity log is to be even more precise and for us to learn what days look like for you.

Why is this useful?

1. It will help you identify your individual patterns of behaviour and mood: everyone is different
2. It will tell us what your week looks like now and we can compare now with your weeks later on
3. Looking closely at your daily routine will give us ideas about where you could add some healthy (non-depressed) activities.

Keeping a record of your activities will enable us to see patterns in how your activities affect your mood.

What do I need to do?

Keep a log of all activities that you do, including those that seem insignificant, like sleeping or watching TV. For now, just do things as you normally would do them. Your task is to write down your activities, trying to be as accurate and as detailed as you can.

Remember, no activity is *no* activity!

Try and include *anything* you do, no matter how small, for example sitting in your room, staring at the wall, lying in bed, waiting for phone to ring.

Rating the activities

We also need to rate the activities. We will use scales applying to the four things that all of us as humans need in order to feel well:

Achievement: Did you get anything out of doing the activity? Did you manage a small task you've been putting off for ages? Score this according to how much achievement it gave you, not how much you think it should have given you!

Closeness: Did the activity make you *feel* closer to anyone, or anything (e.g. a pet, a spiritual presence)? It's the feeling that's important, not whether there were other people actually around.

Enjoyment: How much did you enjoy the activity? How much fun or pleasure did you have doing the activity? Is it something you really like?

Once you've rated each activity on Activity, Closeness and Enjoyment (ACE), have a think about how Important the activity is to you.

Importance: Is the activity something that matters to *you*? Other people's views don't count. We want to find out which activities are most important to you, as these are the ones we want to increase.

Rate each activity on a **0–10 scale** for each of these areas, or however works for you.

Daily mood rating: Think about how you would rate your overall mood for each day, and write this at the bottom of the form. Rate your mood on a 0–10 scale (10 is the best you have ever felt, 0 is the worse you have ever felt and 5 is in the middle).

When should I complete the activity log?

You may choose to record your activities as you do them, or you might prefer to wait until the end of the day and to do it all at once. Whatever works for you is fine, but most people find it's easier to rate them on the day they happened while it's still fresh in their mind. Below you will see activity log examples from Sofia and Jayden to show you how they might look. Don't worry if yours looks different; feel free to record your activities in any way you find useful.

Before next time:

Read over this worksheet

Have a go at filling in the activity log with the activities you do over the next week – remember, you can do this however you feel will work best for you

We will review this together next session to see how you're spending your time.

Other notes from the session:

Activity log example: Sofia

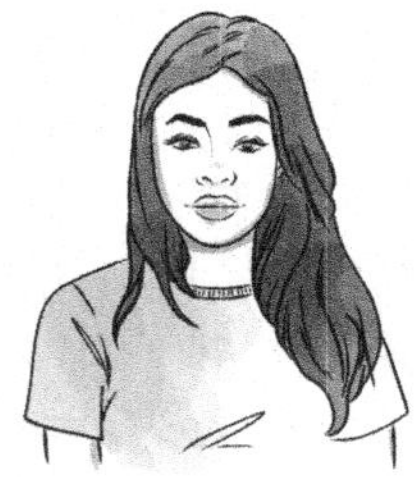

Achievement: 0 = Didn't feel I achieved anything, 10 = Massive achievement!

Closeness: 0 = No closeness (on my own), 10 = Felt really close to someone

Enjoyment: 0 = Hated it! No enjoyment at all, 10 = Loved it, really enjoyed it

Day, date, time	Activity – what I did, who with, and where	Achievement	Closeness	Enjoyment	Important?
Mon 7th March, ~~7am~~ 7.30am	Woke up late	0	0	?	
Mon 7th, 8am	Rushed to get ready for school, forgot homework	1	0	0	
Mon 7th, 8.30am	Bus to school with ~~Harriet~~ Jason and Emma	2	5		
Mon 7th, 8.45–11am	School: Lessons	2	1	0	8
Mon 7th, 11am	Morning break – went to library	4		1	~~4~~ 6
Mon 7th, 11.15-12.30pm	School: Lessons	3	2	1	
Mon 7th, Lunch	Had lunch with Emma, argued	0	1	0	
Mon 7th, Afternoon					
Mon 7th, 4pm	Bus home, sitting alone	0	0	1	
Mon 7th, 5–7pm	Babysat Callum while Mum and Dad at work	2	4	4	
Mon 7th, ~~6.30pm~~ 7pm	Dinner with Mum, Dad and Callum	3	6	5	7
Mon 7th, 8–9pm	Dance class	5	0	2	
Mon 7th, 9–11pm?	Forgot – probably chilling out in room?	DK	DK	DK	DK
Mon 7th, 11–11.45pm	Watched DVD, fell asleep	1	0	3	

Daily mood rating: 0 = Really low, depressed, 10 = Really happy, upbeat

Mon	Tues	Weds	Thurs	Fri	Sat	Sun
4						

Brief activity log example: Jayden

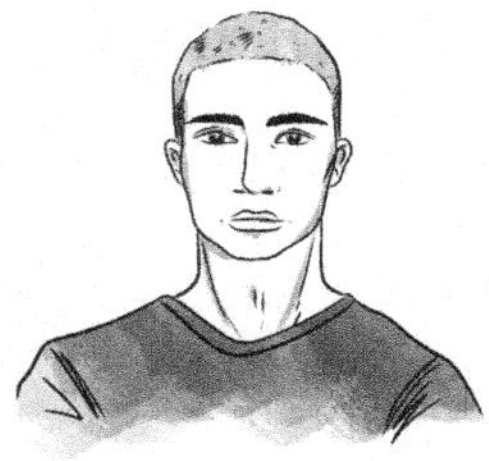

Your mood can be really affected by what you do, where you spend your time, and who you spend it with. Try to record any activities you do (no matter how small or boring you think they are) in the activity log below. Tick each box if you felt the activity gave you *Achievement*, *Closeness* and/or *Enjoyment*. If the activity matters to you, tick the *Important* box.

Day, date, time	Activity – what I did, who with, and where	Achievement	Closeness	Enjoyment	Important?
Mon 7th March, Morning	Slept til midday				
Afternoon	Ate leftovers, lay in bed				
Evening	Played online computer games til 2am	✓		✓	
Tues 8th March, Morning	Got up at 10am, went food shopping with Dad	✓	✓	✓	✓
Afternoon	Watched TV				
Evening	Friend Tom came over, watched funny videos online		✓	✓	✓
Weds 9th March, Morning	Slept til midday				
Afternoon	Played computer games				
Evening	Computer games til midnight			✓	

Source: Adapted from Carol Vivyan's ACE log (www.getselfhelp.co.uk)

Daily mood rating: 0 = Really low, depressed, 10 = Really happy, upbeat

Mon	Tues	Weds	Thurs	Fri	Sat	Sun
3	6	2				

Activity log

Your mood can be really affected by what you do, where you spend your time, and who you spend it with. Try to record any activities you do (no matter how small or boring you think they are) in the activity log below:

Achievement: 0 = Didn't feel I achieved anything, 10 = Massive achievement!

Closeness: 0 = No closeness (on my own), 10 = Felt really close to someone

Enjoyment: 0 = Hated it! No enjoyment at all, 10 = Loved it, really enjoyed it

Day, date, time	Activity – what I did, who with, and where	Achievement	Closeness	Enjoyment	Important?

Source: Adapted from Carol Vivyan's ACE log (www.getselfhelp.co.uk)

Daily mood rating: 0 = Really low, depressed, 10 = Really happy, upbeat

Mon	Tues	Weds	Thurs	Fri	Sat	Sun

Brief activity log

Your mood can be really affected by what you do, where you spend your time, and who you spend it with. Try to record any activities you do (no matter how small or boring you think they are) in the log below. Tick each box if you felt the activity gave you *Achievement*, *Closeness* and/or *Enjoyment*. If the activity matters to you, tick the *Important* box.

Day, date, time	Activity – what I did, who with, and where	Achievement	Closeness	Enjoyment	Important?
Morning					
Afternoon					
Evening					
Morning					
Afternoon					
Evening					
Morning					
Afternoon					
Evening					

Source: Adapted from Carol Vivyan's ACE log (www.getselfhelp.co.uk)

Daily mood rating: 0 = Really low, depressed, 10 = Really happy, upbeat

Mon	Tues	Weds	Thurs	Fri	Sat	Sun

Parent Brief BA Session 1 Worksheet

[Therapist photo here]

Introductions

Therapist's name: **[Full name]**

Contact number: **[Service contact number]**

About depression

Depression is a problem that many teenagers face. Lots of people feel low or sad at some time, but when these feelings don't go away or interfere with everyday life, that's when someone is said to be experiencing depression.

Up to 25% of young people will have experienced depression by the time they are 18.

Depression affects how we feel, our thoughts, our behaviours and our bodies. For some it comes out of the blue, while others have been trying to cope with it for a long time.

When a young person is depressed, you may notice they show a number of changes, including:

- Losing interest or enjoyment, finding things are no longer fun
- Feeling depressed, down, sad or irritable
- Increase or decrease in appetite or weight
- Thinking about death and dying, suicide
- Extreme tiredness, fatigue
- Sleeping too much or not enough
- Difficulties concentrating or making decisions
- Feeling worthless or guilty
- Physical agitation or slowness
- Not wanting to be around people

One of the key differences between depression in adults and in young people is that irritability can be a core symptom of depression in young people. This might come out in their behaviour (e.g. snapping at others, getting easily annoyed at small things) or be something they try hard to contain but feel inside.

Living with a young person who has depression can be very difficult. It is very hard to watch your son or daughter miss out on opportunities, and parents often feel that their child has just changed. It is also usual for parents to feel that they don't know how to help and to feel hopeless. Conflict and family arguments are common, and this can make everyone feel even worse. Do make sure that you look after yourself as well as your family – everyone needs support! If you would like to get extra help for yourself, speak to your own family doctor and find out what is available. A few sources of support are listed below, and at the end of these worksheets there is additional information about books, websites and organizations that you might find useful.

Sometimes parents are not sure about some of the internal changes their child might be experiencing, but often they have noticed some kind of change. It can be helpful to identify what depression symptoms you've noticed, or your child has reported to you.

My child's depression symptoms:

My feelings about my child and their depression:

My sources of support:

Helpful resources for parents

- Parkinson, M. and Reynolds, S. (2015) *Teenage Depression: A CBT Guide for Parents. Help Your Child Beat Their Low Mood*. London: Robinson.
- PAPYRUS, Prevention of Young Suicide, advice and support for people worried about young people dealing with self-harm and emotional distress, https://papyrus-uk.org/im-thinking-about-suicide/ and https://papyrus-uk.org/worried-about-someone
- Young Minds, For Parents, Parents Helpline: 0808 802 5544 (free helpline, open Mon–Fri 9.30am–4pm, or chat online weekdays 11am–1pm), https://youngminds.org.uk/find-help/for-parents

Two teenagers with depression, Jayden and Sofia, will be described throughout the worksheets, to illustrate how depression can affect young people differently, and how the Brief BA approach can be tailored for each individual.

Jayden is 17 years old and was doing a college course in IT but dropped out. He has a Saturday job but hasn't gone recently. He feels down and irritable most of the time, and often snaps at people for no reason. Jayden sleeps a lot during the day as well as at night. He lives with his dad, who has noticed he seems slowed down. Jayden has stopped seeing his friends as he can't be bothered to go out and everything seems like a huge effort. He hates himself and at times has wished he wasn't here.

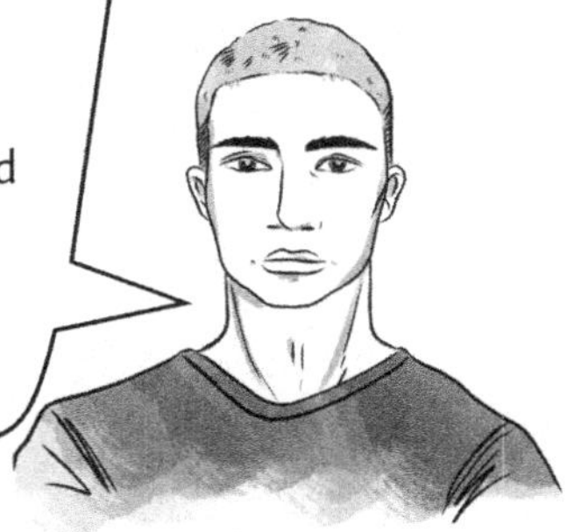

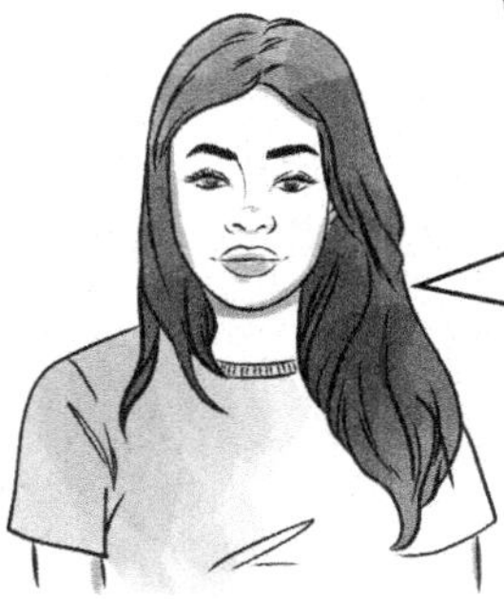

Sofia is 16 years old, and at school studying for her upcoming exams. She feels down most days and cries a lot. Sofia finds it a real struggle to concentrate on homework, and even though she still goes to school and has dance classes twice a week, she feels as if she isn't enjoying anything she does. Sofia finds it hard to get to sleep, and often wakes up in the middle of the night. She has lost her appetite since she started feeling low, and only eats when her mum makes her. She thinks she is a failure and things are never going to improve.

When a teenager is depressed, they may lose motivation to do things, which means:

- They may find it difficult to do even simple things
- They stop doing their normal activities
- They shut off from other people
- They might just 'go through the motions' but not really engage in activities
- They may become inactive, just doing nothing for long periods of time
- They might spend their time online or watching TV shows rather than doing things that you feel they need to get done.

Doing things differently can help your child think and feel differently, even if they find that hard to believe right now.

Depression can be a 'vicious cycle', where the more depressed you feel, the less you want to do (especially the things that take effort or are more difficult). This is understandable given how hard it is to do anything when you're depressed. Unfortunately, the less you do of things that matter, the less 'feel-good' factor you get from life, and the more depressed you feel. Because of this vicious cycle, we find that depression often gets in the way of teenagers building the life that they want.

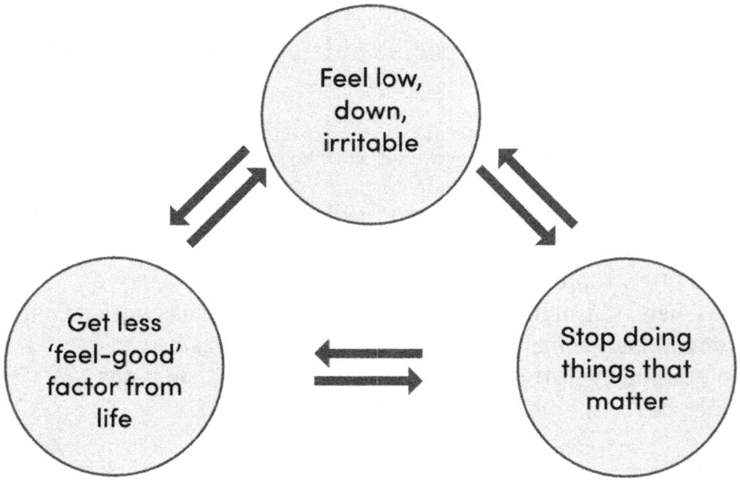

THE VICIOUS CYCLE OF DEPRESSION

What causes depression?

It is difficult to say why someone gets depressed, as everybody is different, and there is no one specific cause for depression. Sometimes the reason may be obvious, sometimes it might not be clear.

Many teenagers can identify 'triggers' to their depression – an event or series of events that happened before they started feeling depressed. It is usually a mixture of things, for example:

- Something difficult happening to them, such as:
  - Parents separating or getting a divorce
  - Friendship difficulties
  - Difficult relationships at home
  - The death of a loved one
  - Relationship break-up
  - Bullying
  - Physical illness
  - Feeling overwhelmed by school or college, failing exams
- Depression can be more likely if a young person is under a lot of stress and has no one to share their worries with
- Depression is more common in people who have experienced long-term stress, including poverty, homelessness, conflict and violence, or abuse
- Depression often runs in families
- There may be biological causes for depression, but these are still unclear and seem to work in combination with life events and adversity.

Jayden started feeling low after struggling with his new college course. Then he broke his ankle and missed a lot of teaching as he couldn't walk far, and dad was working nights so couldn't give him many lifts. When he came back it felt too hard to catch up. His friends are busy with work or college, and his dad struggles with his own depression at times, so he doesn't want to bother him.

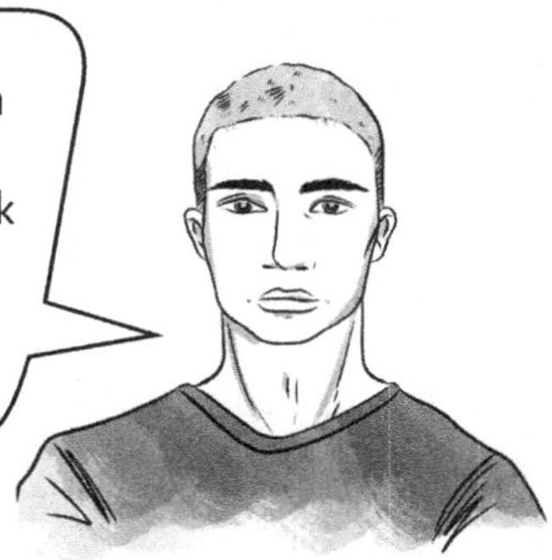

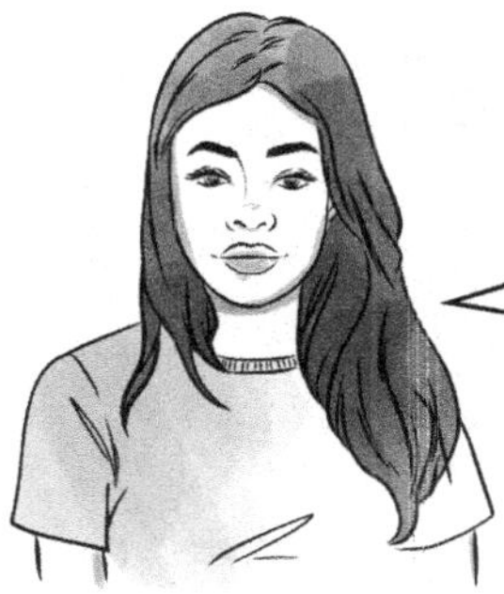

Sofia's low mood started after her gran died last year, and things gradually got worse. She feels as if her parents push her to do a lot of extra studying after school, as well as dance classes. Her best friend has recently got a new girlfriend so Sofia doesn't have anyone to hang out with, which she thinks other people have started to notice.

Possible triggers for my child's depression:

The here and now

Don't worry if you're not sure what might have triggered your child's depression in the first place. The important thing for us to think about together is what's happening now, and what can be changed to help them feel better.

The key to feeling better is not in understanding what caused the depression, but in understanding what is keeping it going.

After 'triggers' or events 'kick off' feelings of depression, it can be hard to figure out ways to feel better. Your child might isolate themselves, not wanting to be around family; they might start spending more time in their room or they might start sleeping a lot or avoiding their friends. This can lead to the vicious cycle described earlier, where feeling low makes them less motivated to do things, but doing less of the important things in life makes them feel even worse.

As everyone is different, together we want to understand what has been happening for your child, to learn more about how we, as a team (you, your child and the therapist), might work together to help improve their mood.

The Brief Behavioural Activation (Brief BA) approach

Brief Behavioural Activation (Brief BA) is based on the idea that your child's ability to feel better has a lot to do with how they live their life on a day-to-day basis.

Brief BA focuses on helping your child develop different patterns of behaviour where they do valued activities every day that help them *break out of this vicious cycle* and start to feel better.

1) **Doing** things differently → **LEADS TO** → 2) **Thinking** and **feeling** differently

BEATING DEPRESSION WITH BRIEF BEHAVIOURAL ACTIVATION

Lots of research has shown BA is an effective way of treating low mood in both adults and young people.

Brief BA is all about increasing activities that are helpful and important to your child, and reducing unhelpful activities.

Role of the Brief BA therapist

Often teenagers with depression have been trying really hard to 'just do it' and feel better on their own, but *changing things on your own isn't easy*. When people are trying to learn new skills like tennis or playing the guitar they often have a coach, teacher or guide. Brief BA involves learning new skills and trying new activities, and your child's therapist will be coaching them on how to do that. The Brief BA therapist's job will be to work closely with your child and you to figure out what activities are right for them, to help them feel better and more in control of their life.

We will work together as a team to help get your child back on track.

Role of parents or other important adults

Many teenagers find it helps to have a coach at home, and that's where parents (or other important adults) can help. By sharing information during and after sessions with parents, it can help parents understand what's going on for their child, what is being covered each week in the sessions, and how parents can help their child make progress. The amount of involvement each teenager wants their parents to have in their treatment varies, but reading these worksheets and being available to support your child in their Brief BA work can make a real difference. We hope this information will also help you feel more confident about how to support your child, and understand how the Brief BA approach might work for them and your family as a whole.

Parents can help their child make the most of this treatment.

Doing work between sessions

To make the most out of what your child and therapist talk about in sessions, it's really important that your child practises in between sessions. Your child will meet their therapist for around one hour a week – that leaves 167 hours outside the sessions! Your child and their therapist will agree specific things to practise between sessions and review this every week to troubleshoot any problems. People do better from treatment if they practise at home! Brief BA is like learning to ride a bike – the more practise your child puts in, the better they will become.

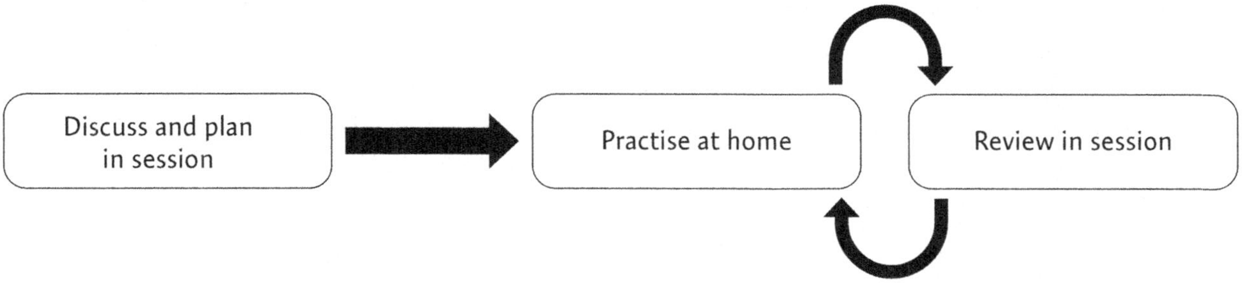

PLAN, PRACTISE, REVIEW CYCLE

Introducing the activity log

After Session 1, your child will be asked to record their activity and their mood every day. Because the main focus of Brief BA treatment is increasing healthy behaviour, it is important to understand how your child is spending each day. Although your child probably feels they already have a good sense of how they spend their time, the purpose of the activity log is to be even more precise, and for us as a team to learn about what they do. Most of us struggle to remember exactly what we've done over the course of a day unless we record it in some way, which is where the activity log comes in.

Why is this useful?

1. It will help us all identify your child's individual patterns of behaviours and moods, as everyone is different
2. It will provide a measure of your child's current activity level, which they can compare with their activity level later in treatment
3. Looking closely at their daily routine might give your child, their therapist and you ideas about how and where your child might want to add some more helpful activities.

Keeping a record of your child's activities will enable them to see patterns in how their activities affect their mood.

By recording their activity and mood your child may notice that they are doing some activities that are not *Important* or *Enjoyable*, or that don't give them a sense of *Achievement* or *Closeness*. Monitoring can help your child figure out what they could stop doing and how to add important and enjoyable activities to each day to help them feel better.

What do they need to do?

To monitor their activities, your child will keep a log of all the activities they do. Their task is to record their activities, trying to be accurate and to include as many activities as they can.

Remember, no activity is *no* activity!

Your child should include *anything* they do, no matter how small, for example sitting in their room, staring at the wall, lying in bed, waiting for the phone to ring. This is different from how we often think about our activities, but this amount of detail will help your child and the Brief BA therapist understand how *exactly* they are spending their time, and where they could make positive changes.

Activity logs can be completed in lots of different ways. The examples we've given are just some suggestions of how activities can be recorded, but there are many others, including everyday diaries or planners, mobile phone apps, electronic record sheets, notebooks, and so on. Your child will explore with their therapist the way they feel is easiest to record their activities, but it may be helpful for you to discuss this with them and consider any ways you could help (e.g. buying them a new notebook to write it in, creating an electronic version together).

Once they have recorded the activity, they will then rate the activity in terms of:

Achievement: Did your child feel they got anything out of doing the activity – for example, did they manage a task they've been putting off for ages? Were they relieved they'd finally done it?

Closeness: Did the activity make them *feel* closer to anyone, or anything (e.g. a pet)? It's the feeling that's important, not whether there were other people actually around (this includes feeling close to a loved one who is no longer here, or getting a sense of spiritual closeness).

Enjoyment: How much did your child enjoy the activity? How much fun or pleasure did they have doing the activity? Is it something they really like?

Once they've rated each activity on Achievement, Closeness and Enjoyment (ACE) on a *0–10 scale* for each, your child should think about how Important the activity is to them.

Importance: Is the activity something that matters to *them*? Other people's views don't count here (even yours, although we know this can be hard!). This is because we want to find out which activities are most important to your child, as these are the ones we want to increase. There is room for discussion about this later if you feel that there are other activities that are also important, but at this stage we want to find out what matters to your child, as this is a route out of depression. They should rate the activity on a 0–10 scale.

Daily mood rating: Your child should think about how they would rate their overall mood for each day, and write this at the bottom of the form. They should rate their mood on a 0–10 scale too. This will help us see the link between your child's activities and their mood.

When should my child complete the activity log?

This is up to them – they may choose to record activities as they do them, or they might prefer to wait until the end of the day to do them all at once. Whatever works for your child is fine, but most people find it's easier to rate them on the day they happened while it's still fresh in their mind. You can help your child to do this in any way that is useful for them, for example reminding them to fill in their activities, completing the log together, helping them remember specific activities they did that day.

How else can I help?

To understand what your child is being asked to do with activity monitoring, you may find it useful to try this yourself. All Brief BA therapists are asked to do the same when starting their training, as it gives a useful insight into what it feels like to monitor how you're spending your time, and how it feels to review this. It may even be an activity you and your child could do together each day (even if they don't feel comfortable sharing with you what they write). Showing them you are willing to do the things being asked of them will give them a greater sense that you're on their side, and that you understand what's involved in Brief BA.

Before next time we would ask your child to:

Read over their worksheets

Have a go at filling in the activity log with the activities as they do them over the week. They can do this in whatever way feels manageable, and will have talked with their Brief BA therapist about what this might look like

This will be reviewed in the next session.

Below are some examples of activity logs completed by Sofia and Jayden, the young people we discussed earlier. As you can see, Sofia has completed her log very thoroughly, rating every activity on Activity, Closeness, Enjoyment and Importance. Jayden has chosen to tick the boxes instead. Both are absolutely fine. It's also fine to record activity logs using the computer or apps, and your son or daughter can be as creative as they like and design their own activity logs if they prefer.

Activity log example: Sofia

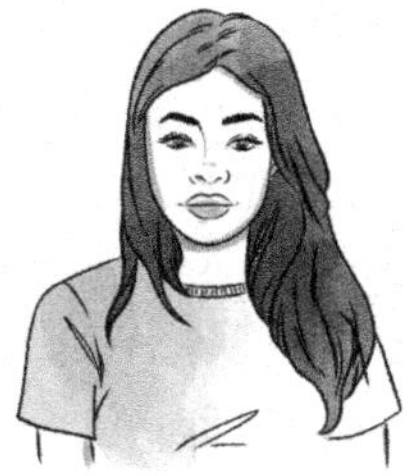

Achievement: 0 = Didn't feel I achieved anything, 10 = Massive achievement!

Closeness: 0 = No closeness (on my own), 10 = Felt really close to someone

Enjoyment: 0 = Hated it! No enjoyment at all, 10 = Loved it, really enjoyed

Day, date, time	Activity – what I did, who with, and where	Achievement	Closeness	Enjoyment	Important?
Mon 7th March, ~~7am~~ 7.30am	Woke up late	0	0	?	
Mon 7th, 8am	Rushed to get ready for school, forgot homework	1	0	0	
Mon 7th, 8.30am	Bus to school with ~~Harriet~~ Jason and Emma	2	5		
Mon 7th, 8.45–11am	School: Lessons	2	1	0	8
Mon 7th, 11am	Morning break – went to library	4		1	~~4~~ 6
Mon 7th, 11.15-12.30pm	School: Lessons	3	2	1	
Mon 7th, Lunch	Had lunch with Emma, argued	0	1	0	
Mon 7th, Afternoon					
Mon 7th, 4pm	Bus home, sitting alone	0	0	1	
Mon 7th, 5–7pm	Babysat Callum while Mum and Dad at work	2	4	4	
Mon 7th, ~~6.30pm~~ 7pm	Dinner with Mum, Dad and Callum	3	6	5	7
Mon 7th, 8–9pm	Dance class	5	0	2	
Mon 7th, 9–11pm?	Forgot – probably chilling out in room?	DK	DK	DK	DK
Mon 7th, 11–11.45pm	Watched DVD, fell asleep	1	0	3	

Daily mood rating: 0 = Really low, depressed, 10 = Really happy, upbeat

Mon	Tues	Weds	Thurs	Fri	Sat	Sun
4						

Brief activity log example: Jayden

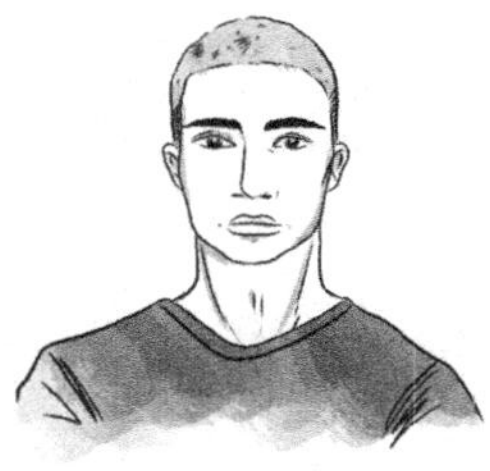

Your mood can be really affected by what you do, where you spend your time, and who you spend it with. Try to record any activities you do (no matter how small or boring you think they are) in the log below. Tick each box if you felt the activity gave you *Achievement*, *Closeness*, and/or *Enjoyment*. If the activity matters to you, tick the *Important* box.

Day, date, time	**Activity – what I did, who with, and where**	**Achievement**	**Closeness**	**Enjoyment**	**Important?**
Mon 7th March, Morning	Slept til midday				
Afternoon	Ate leftovers, lay in bed				
Evening	Played online computer games til 2am	✓		✓	
Tues 8th March, Morning	Got up at 10am, went food shopping with Dad	✓	✓	✓	✓
Afternoon	Watched TV				
Evening	Friend Tom came over, watched funny videos online		✓	✓	✓
Weds 9th March, Morning	Slept til midday				
Afternoon	Played computer games				
Evening	Computer games til midnight			✓	

Source: Adapted from Carol Vivyan's ACE log (www.getselfhelp.co.uk)

Daily mood rating: 0 = Really low, depressed, 10 = Really happy, upbeat

Mon	Tues	Weds	Thurs	Fri	Sat	Sun
3	6	2				

Activity log

Your mood can be really affected by what you do, where you spend your time, and who you spend it with. Try to record any activities you do (no matter how small or boring you think they are) in the log below:

Achievement: 0 = Didn't feel I achieved anything, 10 = Massive achievement!

Closeness: 0 = No closeness (on my own), 10 = Felt really close to someone

Enjoyment: 0 = Hated it! No enjoyment at all, 10 = Loved it, really enjoyed it

Day, date, time	Activity – what I did, who with, and where	Achievement	Closeness	Enjoyment	Important?

Source: Adapted from Carol Vivyan's ACE log (www.getselfhelp.co.uk)

Daily mood rating: 0 = Really low, depressed, 10 = Really happy, upbeat

Mon	Tues	Weds	Thurs	Fri	Sat	Sun

Brief activity log

Your mood can be really affected by what you do, where you spend your time, and who you spend it with. Try to record any activities you do (no matter how small or boring you think they are) in the log below. Tick each box if you felt the activity gave you *Achievement*, *Closeness*, and/or *Enjoyment*. If the activity matters to you, tick the *Important* box.

Day, date, time	Activity – what I did, who with, and where	Achievement	Closeness	Enjoyment	Important?
Morning					
Afternoon					
Evening					
Morning					
Afternoon					
Evening					
Morning					
Afternoon					
Evening					

Source: Adapted from Carol Vivyan's ACE log (www.getselfhelp.co.uk)

Daily mood rating: 0 = Really low, depressed, 10 = Really happy, upbeat

Mon	Tues	Weds	Thurs	Fri	Sat	Sun

Stay positive!

Parenting a depressed teenager can be *really* hard work. It might feel that they do very little, and are not trying to keep up with things they used to enjoy. It can be frustrating to see them withdraw from things you think would help them.

However, key symptoms of depression include a lack of interest and pleasure in things they used to enjoy, fatigue and feelings of worthlessness. Understandably, it's hard to be able to do things if you are struggling with these symptoms.

What can you do?

The vicious cycle of depression is maintained by life being less rewarding for your teenager. 'Rewards' means anything positive: achieving something, feeling close to others, simply having fun or getting positive feedback from others. By increasing praise, encouragement and other rewards as well as reducing negative interactions with your depressed teenager, you can really make a difference by making their life more rewarding.

By giving your teenager positive encouragement, you are making their life more rewarding.

Positive encouragement is the best way to show your teenager you are noticing their efforts, however small. It is also helping to redress the imbalance in the vicious cycle of depression – depressed teenagers often don't have opportunities to get rewarding contacts with others. Every time you praise or encourage your teenager, you are helping to redress the balance.

Redressing the balance: Making life more rewarding.

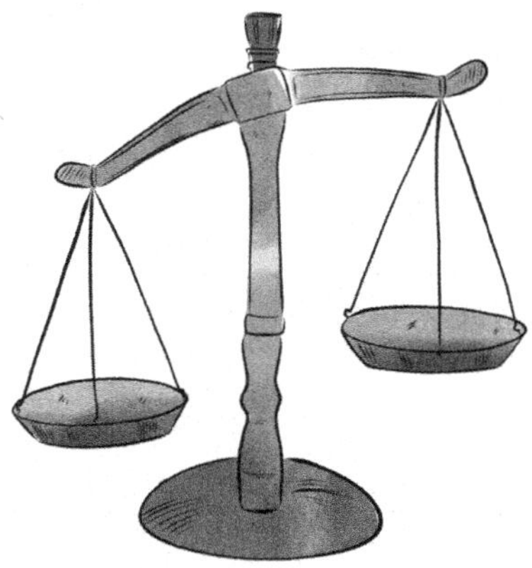

Even if your teenager doesn't look as if they're trying hard, they're fighting an ongoing battle against their negative feelings. Every tiny step is progress in the right direction, and to them it may feel like a marathon!

Sometimes parents have understandably tried to help their teenager by reducing demands on them, not wanting to be seen as nagging or adding to their problems. In some ways this is helpful to reduce conflict. However, we want to help them get back into healthy, non-depressed behaviours, so make sure any reduction in demands is matched by an increase in praise for active behaviours and efforts at doing things that may be hard but that are helpful for their wellbeing.

Key tips for staying positive

Do:

- Look for the positive and praise this at every opportunity
- Recognize the effort it takes for your teenager to do even small things when they are depressed
- Use verbal and non-verbal (hugs, smiles) ways of showing them you're pleased
- Give your teenager your time and attention when they are making an effort to engage in non-depressed behaviour (e.g. being active, helping out at home, being sociable, taking care of themselves)
- Be inventive in your positivity: send a text, leave a post-it, give them a funny card or picture
- Seek support from others to help you stay positive and calm.

Don't:

- Be critical: criticism can feel even more painful when you're already feeling critical of yourself
- Put up barriers to them doing activities unless you have a good reason
- Show hostility in your words or actions
- Praise depressed behaviours (e.g. avoidance or withdrawal – staying in, avoiding parties).

REWARDING PHRASES

'Thanks for helping'	'I'm impressed'	'I can see how hard you're trying'
'You're being a really good friend'	'Well done for being responsible'	'Fantastic!'
'That must have taken a lot of effort, well done'	'I love you'	'I know you can do it'
'I've got faith in you'	'That's a great idea'	'Thank you for being considerate'
'You're very important to me'	'Let's just have a go together, shall we?'	'Keep trying'
'You're nearly there'	'I'm really proud of you'	'That was really nice of you'

Things I'd say to be rewarding, in my own words:

Brief BA Session 2 Checklist

ID/Client initials:

Date:

Brief BA Session 2 Checklist *Young person seen alone for majority of the session*	
Complete?	**Task**
	Audio/video recorder on
	Anything in particular to make time for today? Details:
	Complete ROMs: • Young person symptom questionnaire (e.g. RCADS Depression Subscale + Risk Q, or full RCADS if not done recently) • Young person functioning/quality of life questionnaire (e.g. ORS) • Parent report of young person symptom questionnaire (e.g. RCADS Depression Subscale + Risk Q, or full RCADS if not done recently) • Parent report of young person functioning/quality of life questionnaire (e.g. ORS)
	Risk discussion
	Feed back full young person and parent RCADS scores from Session 1 (if not done previously), what the scores mean for age/sex of client
	Review goal progress (if appropriate)
	Bridge from last time (suggestions of points raised last time to revisit):
	Review activity log
	(If needed, troubleshoot completion of activity log)
	Check understanding and engagement with Brief BA approach
	Recap Brief BA model (use young person example if possible)
	Introduce values
	Agree homework: complete activity log
	Photocopy young person's completed session worksheets
	Give young person session worksheets to take away
	Give parent session worksheets to take away
	Confirm next session date, time, location
	Young person session feedback questionnaire (e.g. SRS)

After Session 2	
Complete?	**Task**
	Upload audio/video recording and delete from device
	Score young parent and parent ROMs (if not done in session)
	Outcome electronic diary appointment (if applicable)
	Electronic or paper session record: ROMs, risk, attendees, content, homework, next appointment
	Upload completed session worksheets and ROMs to electronic records (if applicable)
	Diary appointment for next session
	Prepare to discuss in supervision
	Book room for next session

Young Person Brief BA Session 2 Worksheet

Top tips for completing the activity log

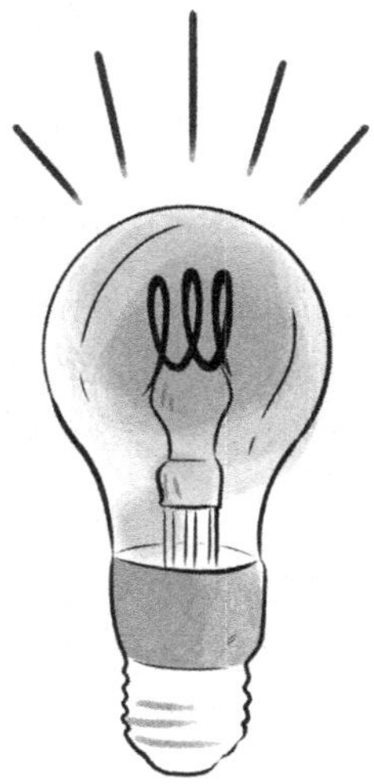

- ✓ You will remember more activities if you get into the habit of writing them down
- ✓ If it's easier, keep your logs super brief, e.g. 'lunch with Sam', 'did homework'
- ✓ You can also just tick A, C, E, or I boxes rather than using the 0–10 rating if you prefer, or any other way you like
- ✓ It's okay if it's not all complete; just do as much as you can
- ✓ Put the activity log somewhere you'll see it regularly – e.g. on your bedroom wall, by the computer, on the fridge
- ✓ Try setting a reminder on your phone for a time you're likely to be free (e.g. after dinner)
- ✓ If you're somewhere where it's not easy to fill in the log, send a text or email to yourself
- ✓ Put a post-it somewhere you can't miss – on your mirror? Next to the light switch?
- ✓ Ask your parents to remind you.

Remember, *this has got to work for you*; you can record it however you want – on your phone, on a calendar, on scrap pieces of paper. We just need to make sure we can review it in our sessions, as *it is important to the Brief BA approach.*

Introducing values

Your values are 'what matters to you'. We will help you identify what matters to you, and then increase activities that fit with your values. This will challenge depressed behaviour. It will help you feel better and able to get on with your life.

In other words, we are going to teach you a different way of organizing your days that will make it more likely that you will experience more positive experiences and reward from everyday life.

It's hard to feel depressed when you are regularly doing activities that are valuable, enjoyable and important to you.

As everyone is different, we want to understand what has been happening for you, to learn more about how we might work together to improve your mood.

Jayden doesn't do much with his time except sleep and play computer games. He stopped playing basketball when he broke his ankle, and can't be bothered to go back to his local club, even though his ankle is better now. He hasn't turned up to his Saturday job twice in a row, as it just feels like too much effort.

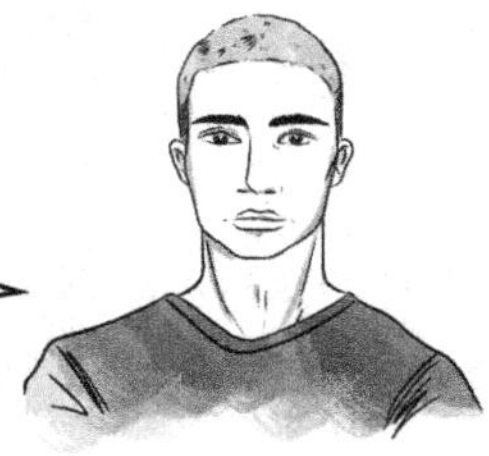

Many young people with depression feel tired and lack the motivation to do various activities, thinking that once they have more energy and feel more positively, they'll be able to do more.

We take the opposite approach in Brief BA. Behaviour is changed first as a *way* to increase energy and motivation, as well as helping you feel better.

Changing behaviour is one of the easiest ways to break the vicious cycle of depression, to help you feel better over time. This won't happen overnight (unfortunately); it can take a bit of time to get working, but when it does work, it is very effective!

How Brief BA breaks the depression cycle

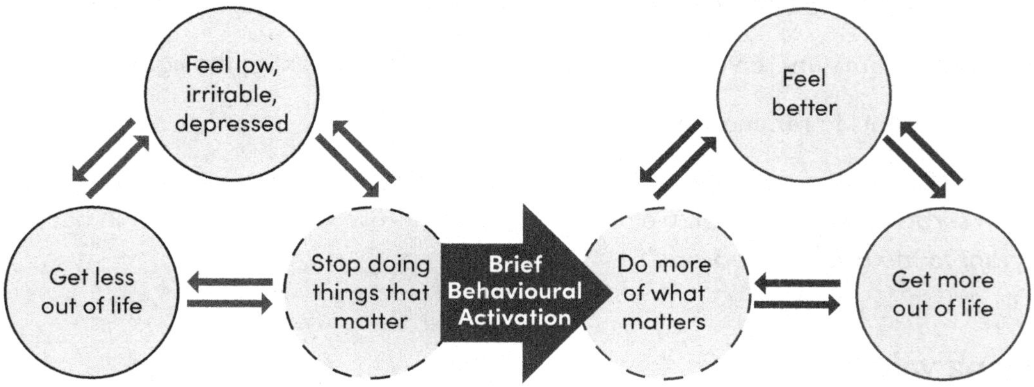

THE BRIEF BA MODEL

At the moment you probably aren't doing much that really matters to you. By deciding what matters to you and doing more of this we will start a positive cycle of activity. You will get more out of life and start to feel better. Then you will be able to do even more of what matters to you.

What if I am already doing a lot but still feel down?

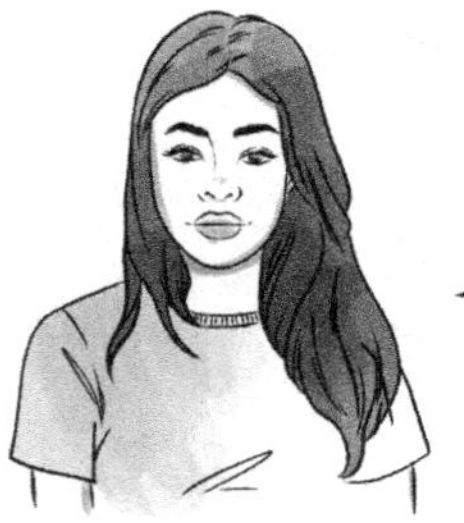

Sofia does a lot each week – she has school every day, then homework and revision, plus dance classes, babysitting her brother and piano lessons. Sofia feels as if she is always busy, but she's not really connecting with the things she does. She feels pushed to do things that her parents want her to do, not what she wants to do.

It is possible to be active but still be depressed. This can happen if you're doing lots of things that you don't feel are important to you, or things you feel pushed to do by others. For example, a lot of teenagers work hard at school or college, but don't do much to look after themselves, do interests or hobbies, or make time for the people who matter to them.

It is important not just to do more, but to do more things that fit with what is important to you.

That's why we want to work together to understand exactly how you're spending your time at the moment, and how this fits with what's important to you.

It could be that we find some important areas of your life aren't getting much attention, so you decide these are the areas to focus on when increasing activities. Sometimes, this may mean doing less of other activities that are not important or meaningful for you. We can discuss this together before making any changes, but if you feel you want to get started, go ahead!

Before next time:

Read through these pages and add them to Session 1 in your folder

If possible, share the session work with your parents

Keep filling in your activity log: try to put as much detail as possible, and rate each activity for Achievement, Enjoyment, Closeness and Importance

We will review your activity log next session.

Other notes from the session:

Parent Brief BA Session 2 Worksheet

Completing the activity log

Hopefully your child managed to complete some kind of activity log, but we know that some teenagers find it hard. If your child found it difficult, we need to understand why, so we can work on this.

What if they already know how they spend their time?

- Writing it down can help us think about these things together in session, and look at the ratings that your child has given each activity
- Your child will remember more activities if they get into the habit of writing them down. This gives more information to draw on in Brief BA
- A lot of young people are surprised by patterns they notice on the activity log, and find it helps them get a real understanding of how certain patterns lead to more depressed feelings while others lead to more positive feelings.

What if it's too much effort for them to fill in the activity log?

- Encourage your child to keep their logs as brief as possible, e.g. 'lunch with Sam', 'did homework'
- Talk with your child about what might help (including you supporting them with filling it in)
- If giving a 0–10 rating is too hard, they can just put a tick if the activity gave your child a sense of Achievement, Closeness, and/or Enjoyment, and if they felt it was Important to them
- If your child finds it hard to decide if it's an Important activity, they can put the rest down and we can talk about this in the session
- Talk about ways to make this easier for them, linking to things that generally help them when a task is too big.

What if they (and I) keep forgetting?

- Put the activity log somewhere your child will see it regularly – e.g. on their bedroom wall, by the computer, on the fridge
- Try setting a reminder on your phone to remind your child to complete it – at a time they are likely to be free (e.g. after dinner)
- If your child is somewhere where it's not easy to fill in the log, they can send a text or email to you or themselves
- Put a post-it note somewhere your child can't miss – on their mirror? Next to the light switch? On their laptop?
- Try setting this as a task for you to do as well as them, so both of you are trying to remember

- Use these and other ways to remind yourself to remind your child: what helps you to remember other things you or they need to do every day?
- Remember, this has got to work for your child; they can record it however they want – on their phone, on a calendar or on scrap pieces of paper. We just need to make sure we can review it in our sessions, as it is really important to the Brief BA approach.

Brief BA is all about increasing activities that are helpful and important to your child, and reducing unhelpful activities.

Introducing values

We will help your child identify what is important to them and then help them to increase healthy behaviour that fits with this and challenges depressed behaviour. As they do more activities that are important to them, they will feel more positive and develop greater self-esteem and confidence.

In other words, we are going to teach your child a different way of organizing their days that will make it more likely that they will experience more positive experiences and reward from life every day. When there are *regular*, *stable* and *diverse* sources of reward in a young person's life, they are 'filling up the reward tank' so will feel better and have more resources to cope with life's problems.

It's hard for people to feel depressed when they are regularly doing activities that are valuable, enjoyable and important to them.

As everyone is different, we want to understand what has been happening for your child, to learn more about how we might work together to improve your child's mood.

Jayden doesn't do much with his time except sleep and play computer games. He stopped playing basketball when he broke his ankle, and he can't be bothered to go back to his local club even though his ankle is better now. He hasn't turned up to his Saturday job twice in a row, as it just feels like too much effort. He struggles to even be bothered to get dressed some days.

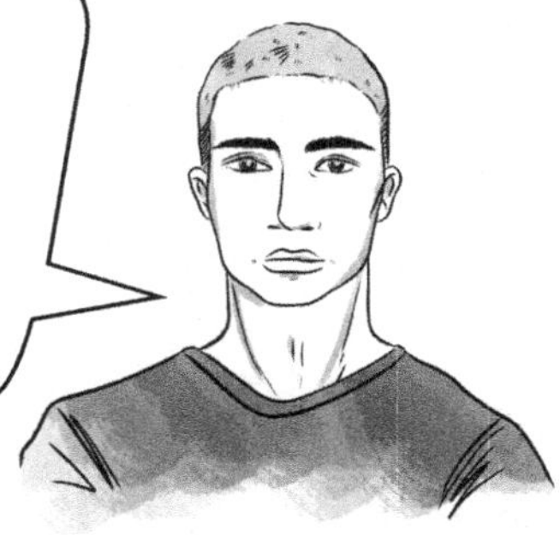

Many young people with depression feel tired and lack the motivation to do various activities, thinking that once they have more energy and feel more positively, they'll be able to do more.

The opposite approach is taken in this treatment. In Brief BA, we aim to change behaviour first as a *way* to increase energy and motivation, as well as helping them feel better.

How Brief BA can break the depression cycle

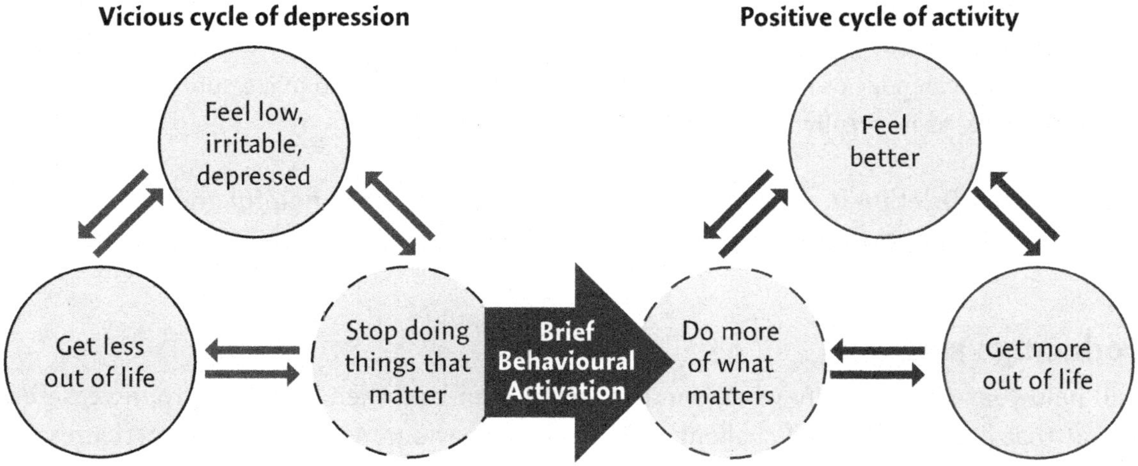

THE BRIEF BA MODEL

Changing behaviour is an effective way to break the vicious cycle of depression and to help your child start thinking more positively and feel better.

This won't happen overnight (unfortunately); it is a treatment that can take bit of time to get working, but when it does work, it is very effective!

By looking at the activities your child is doing and working together to make sure they are enjoyable and important, we can then kick-start a positive cycle of activity. This will have a knock-on effect on how they feel. You can help with this by encouraging them to record how they spend their time, and, if they are happy to, talking about how this fits with what matters to them.

It can help to be curious about *why* your child finds activities important, even if you personally might not agree that a specific activity is valuable. Showing them you are interested in their view is important. Even if you share their opinion on valued and important activities, it's surprising how people can get value from the same activity for very different reasons. Exploring this with your child will help you find out more about them and what they find important.

What if my child is already doing a lot but still feels down?

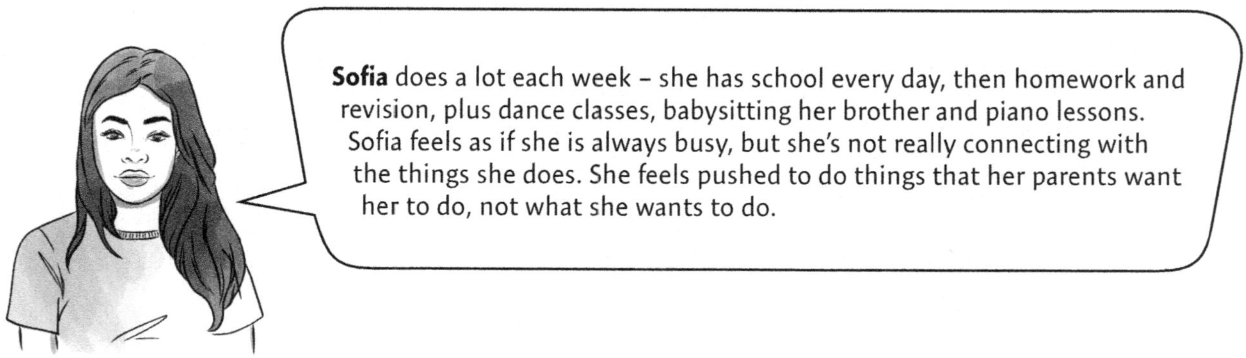

It is possible to be active but still be depressed. This can happen if your child is doing lots of things that they don't feel are important to them, or feel pushed to do by others. For example, a lot of teenagers work hard at school or college, but don't do much to look after themselves, do interests or hobbies, or make time for the people who matter to them. Sometimes this feeling of being pushed to do certain activities might reflect how others are acting towards a young person, while other times it can be an expectation that the young person has rather than what is actually happening.

It is important for your child not just to do more, but to do more things that fit with what is important to them.

That's why we want to work together to understand exactly how your child is spending their time at the moment, and how this fits with what's important to them.

We may find some important areas of your child's life that aren't getting much attention. If so, they might decide these are the areas to focus on when increasing activities. Sometimes, this may mean doing less of other activities that are not as important or meaningful for your child, but we will discuss this together before making any changes. Often this also fits with what parents think is important, but sometimes the balance needs to be fixed.

If you are unsure about possible changes to your child's routine or activities, we suggest talking to your child about why they feel this would be useful to help them feel better. You should also speak to their therapist if you have any concerns. Remember, you are part of the team working to help your child, so your view is important.

Before next time we would ask your child to:

Read through these pages and add them to Session 1 in their folder

If possible, share the session work with you, their parents

Keep filling in their activity log: trying to put as much detail as possible, and rating each activity for Achievement, Enjoyment, Closeness and Importance

We will review your child's activity log next session.

Brief BA Session 3 Checklist

ID/Client initials:

Date:

Brief BA Session 3 Checklist *Young person seen alone for majority of the session*	
Complete?	**Task**
	Audio/video recorder on
	Anything in particular to make time for today? Details:
	Complete ROMs: • Young person symptom questionnaire (e.g. RCADS Depression Subscale + Risk Q, or full RCADS if not done recently) • Young person functioning/quality of life questionnaire (e.g. ORS) • Parent report of young person symptom questionnaire (e.g. RCADS Depression Subscale + Risk Q, or full RCADS if not done recently) • Parent report of young person functioning/quality of life questionnaire (e.g. ORS)
	Risk discussion
	Review goal progress (if appropriate)
	Bridge from last time (suggestions of points raised last time to revisit):
	Review activity monitoring (including troubleshooting if not completed activity log)
	Introduce life areas, values and activities (LAVA) worksheet with focus on values
	Identify one target activity
	Agree homework: complete activity log, fill in the LAVA worksheet, complete one target activity
	Photocopy young person's completed session worksheets
	Give young person session worksheets to take away
	Give parent session worksheets to take away
	Confirm next session date, time, location
	Young person session feedback questionnaire (e.g. SRS)

After Session 3	
Complete?	**Task**
	Upload audio/video recording and delete from device
	Score young person and parent ROMs (if not done in session)
	Outcome electronic diary appointment (if applicable)
	Electronic or paper session record: ROMs, risk, attendees, content, homework, next appointment
	Upload completed session worksheets and ROMs to electronic records (if applicable)
	Diary appointment for next session
	Prepare to discuss in supervision
	Book room for next session

Young Person Brief BA Session 3 Worksheet

Activity log: What have I noticed?

What stood out?

What activities were helpful for my mood?

What was missing that I would like to see?

What do I want to change?

What if I'm not doing anything fun or important?

Often depressed teenagers withdraw from activities that are important to them and end up spending lots of their time doing activities that don't score highly on any of the key factors – *Achievement*, *Closeness*, *Enjoyment* and *Importance*.

Jayden's activity log shows that he only does a few main activities each day, and is particularly low on *Achievement* and *Closeness*. The only activities he rates as *Enjoyable* are playing computer games, but he doesn't feel this really matters to him. He has stopped doing a lot of things since he started feeling depressed, and spends most of his time in bed. Sometimes he doesn't leave the house, shower or even get dressed.

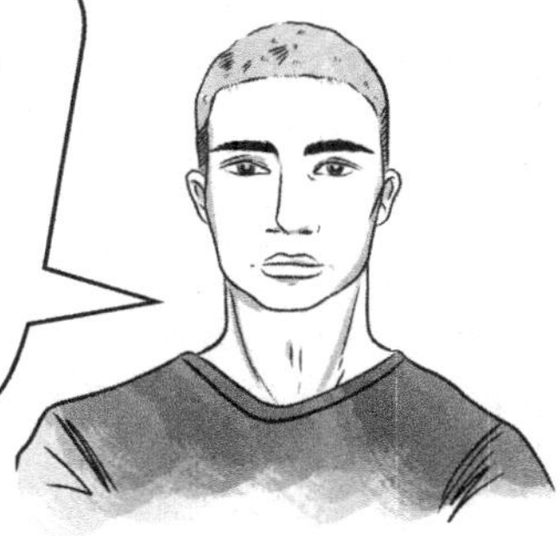

What if I'm doing lots of important things?

Some teenagers can end up spending lots of time working, helping others, and doing things that are expected of them, but don't spend time looking after themselves or just doing things for fun.

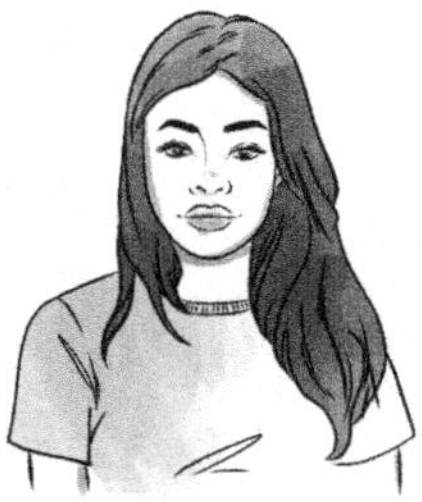

Sofia's activity log shows that she does lots of activities each week that she does not feel are *Important*, but other people do. Even though lots of her activities involve other people, she still does not get a feeling of *Closeness* from them, or *Enjoyment*. She does so many of these activities she doesn't feel she has time to do other things that she would enjoy more.

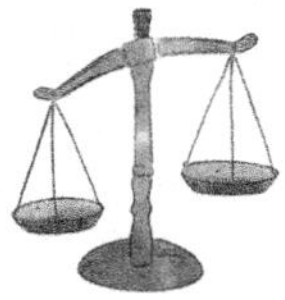

It is important to get a balance of activities, so all areas of your life are being looked after.

Introducing life areas and values

Part of Brief BA involves thinking about the most important areas in your life, and what values are important in each.

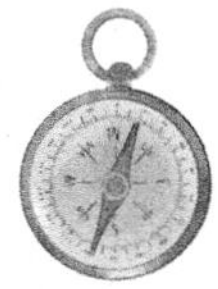

Values are how you would like to approach each area of life, and what really matters to you.

Values give you a sense of purpose and meaning. They are a bit like a compass – showing you the direction you want to go in, rather than the destination.

No one else can tell you what your values are or what they should be; they are personal to you.

To make it easier to think about values relating to different aspects of your life (to find out how balanced things are at the moment), life areas can be grouped into three broad categories:

- *Me* (hobbies/fun, physical health, looking after myself)
- *Things that matter* (education or work, things I need to do, the bigger picture)
- *People who matter* (family, friends, important others).

On the next page is a life areas and values worksheet to help you and your therapist work out what matters to you – what your values are. These are personal to you and might not be the same as your parents' or friends' values. You will also see how Sofia and Jayden filled this in – it might give you some ideas, but remember that your values are *your* values, not someone else's. Try to find values in each of the main areas, but you don't need to fill in all the boxes, and you can have more than one value in each box.

When we know what *your* values are, we will plan activities that will help you live according to your values – activities that will matter to you. It is important to aim for a balance of activities across your different values.

Life areas and values

Me	Things that matter	People who matter
Hobbies/fun How would you like to spend your free time? What is fun for you?	**Education or work** What do you want to achieve? What do you want to learn about?	**Family** What kind of relationships do you want with your family?
Physical health How do you want to look after your body?	**Everyday stuff** What do you need to do?	**Friends** What kind of friend do you want to be? Who with?
Looking after myself What do you do for *you*? What relaxes you? What helps you?	**The bigger picture** Are you religious? Do you care about environmental issues? Politics? Something else?	**Important other(s)** What kind of a relationship do you want? What qualities? Who with?

Life areas and values example: Sofia

Me	Things that matter	People who matter
Hobbies/fun Keep up to date with music and films	**Education or work** Do well at school Study to become a vet	**Family** Be a kind sister Be patient with my dad
Physical health Eat healthily Keep active	**Everyday stuff** Be organized	**Friends** Be a caring friend
Looking after myself Get enough sleep Make time for me	**The bigger picture** Go to church Care about animal welfare	**Important other(s)** Make an effort with Gran

Life areas and values example: Jayden

Me	Things that matter	People who matter
Hobbies/fun	**Education or work** Improve my career prospects	**Family** Help Dad out Spend time with my family
Physical health Get fit again	**Everyday stuff** Get started on things	**Friends** Don't be a stranger to my mates
Looking after myself Spend time outside	**The bigger picture** Help out in the community Give something back	**Important other(s)** Think about other people's feelings

Valued activities

Valued activities are things you can do to live according to your values. They are useful to think about because:

- Without the activities that help you live according to your values, values are just words and ideas, and not a reality
- Activities are things you actually can do as opposed to something you think or feel, so they are easier to monitor and plan
- There can be more than one activity you can do to fit with a value.

Activities are specific ways to head in the direction of your values.

Value: Be a caring friend

Activity: Call Liz once a week and ask about her college course

Activity: Text Seb every day while he is off sick

Activity: Help Jo with her media assignment

MY TARGET ACTIVITY THIS WEEK:

Activity:

Day/time I can do this activity:

Where I can do this activity:

Anything that might get in the way:

How I make sure it happens:

Before next time:

Fill in the activity log over the week

Look through and edit your values worksheet. We will review these next session to see how you got on

Try one small valued activity this week.

Parent Brief BA Session 3 Worksheet

Activity log: What kind of activities is your child doing? Are there things they are not doing that they used to, or that you think might be helpful to do?

Do they score high on *Achievement, Closeness, Enjoyment* and are they *Important*? Or none of these things?

What if my child is not doing much that's meaningful to them?

Often depressed teenagers find themselves spending very little time doing activities that are enjoyable. Some people withdraw from activities that are important to them and end up spending lots of their time doing activities that don't score highly on any of the key factors – *Achievement, Closeness, Enjoyment* and *Importance*.

Jayden's activity log shows that he only does a few main activities each day, and is particularly low on *Achievement* and *Closeness*. The only activities he rates as *Enjoyable* are playing computer games, but he doesn't feel this really matters to him. He has stopped doing a lot of things since he started feeling depressed, and spends most of his time in bed. He doesn't always shower, get dressed or leave the house.

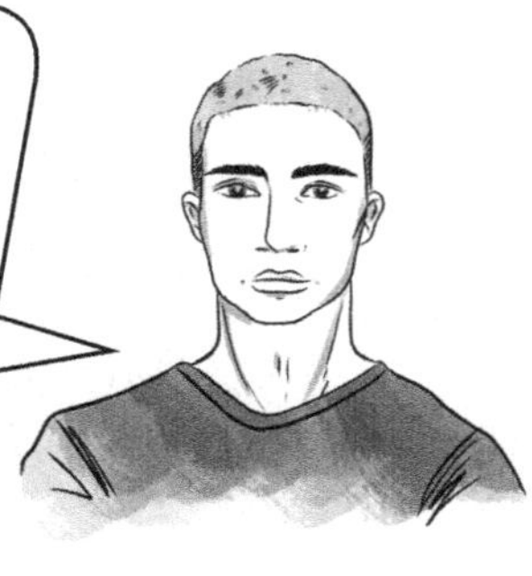

What if my child is doing lots of important things?

Other depressed teenagers find they're doing many *important* activities (e.g. school or college work), but hardly any that are *enjoyable*. They might also find that the activities they are doing are important to other people (e.g. parents, teachers), but not very important to them. This is something to look out for when you're thinking about what you would like your child to be doing more of – activities that are meaningful to them are the ones that will improve their mood.

Some teenagers can end up spending lots of time working, helping others, and doing things that are expected of them, but don't spend time looking after themselves or just doing things for fun. While many of these activities might be important to some extent, the balance needs to be right, and having fun, relaxing and feeling close to others are also key to our mood and wellbeing.

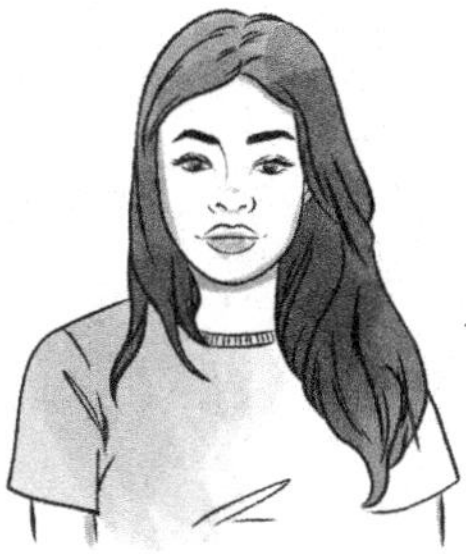

Sofia's activity log shows that she does lots of activities each week that she does not feel are personally *Important*, but other people do. Even though lots of her activities involve other people, she still does not get a feeling of *Closeness* from them, or *Enjoyment*. She does so many of these activities she doesn't feel she has time to do other things that she would enjoy more.

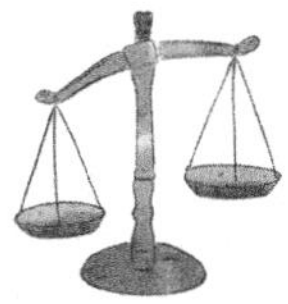

It is important to get a balance of activities, so that all areas of your child's life are being looked after.

Introducing life areas and values

Part of Brief BA involves thinking about the most important areas in your child's life, and what values they have across different life areas.

What do you mean, values?

Values are how you would like to approach each area of life, and what really matters to you.

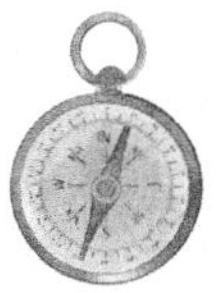

Values can be thought of as how you'd want other people to describe you.

Values give you a sense of purpose and meaning. They are a bit like a compass – showing you the direction you want to go in, rather than the destination.

No one else can tell you what your child's values are or what they should be; they are personal to them.

To make it easier to think about values relating to different aspects of your child's life (to find out how balanced things are at the moment), life areas can be grouped into three broad categories:

- *Me* (individual values linked to hobbies/fun, physical health, looking after themselves)
- *Things that matter* (wider aspects that are important to them including education/work, things they need to do, the bigger picture)
- *People who matter* (interpersonal values around family, friends, and important others).

Below is a life areas and values worksheet we will use with your child to help identify their values. The boxes provide general suggestions. Next you will see the life areas and values worksheet completed by Sofia and Jayden, showing what they thought mattered most to them.

Life areas and values

Me	Things that matter	People who matter
Hobbies/fun How would you like to spend your free time? What is fun for you?	**Education or work** What do you want to achieve? What do you want to learn about?	**Family** What kind of relationships do you want with your family?
Physical health How do you want to look after your body?	**Everyday stuff** What do you need to do?	**Friends** What kind of friend do you want to be? Who with?
Looking after myself What do you do for *you*? What relaxes you? What helps you?	**The bigger picture** Are you religious? Do you care about environmental issues? Politics? Something else?	**Important other(s)** What kind of a relationship do you want? What qualities? Who with?

Life areas and values example: Sofia

Me	Things that matter	People who matter
Hobbies/fun Keep up to date with music and films	**Education or work** Do well at school Study to become a vet	**Family** Be a kind sister Be patient with my dad
Physical health Eat healthily Keep active	**Everyday stuff** Be organized	**Friends** Be a caring friend
Looking after myself Get enough sleep Make time for me	**The bigger picture** Go to church Care about animal welfare	**Important other(s)** Make an effort with Gran

Life areas and values example: Jayden

Me	Things that matter	People who matter
Hobbies/fun	**Education or work** Improve my career prospects	**Family** Help Dad out Spend time with my family
Physical health Get fit again	**Everyday stuff** Get started on things	**Friends** Don't be a stranger to my mates
Looking after myself Spend time outside	**The bigger picture** Help out in the community Give something back	**Important other(s)** Think about other people's feelings

Why think about values?

Doing activities that are important to us can help to make us feel better. By thinking about our values we can then make sure we can identify activities that help us to work towards that value. For example, if one of your values is 'To be a caring friend', there are many different activities that could help work towards that – these are valued activities. Valued activities are likely to help improve mood more than non-valued activities, because they directly link to things that are important to you, and so give you that 'feel-good' factor.

Valued activities

Valued activities are things your child can do, to live according to their values. They are useful to think about because:

- Without the activities that help your child live according to their values, values are just words and ideas, and not a reality
- Activities are things you can actually do as opposed to something you think or feel, so they are *easier to monitor and plan*
- There can be more than one activity you can do to fit with a value.

Activities are specific ways to head in the direction of your child's values.

Value: Be a caring friend
Activity: Call Liz once a week and ask about her college course
Activity: Text Seb every day while he is off sick
Activity: Help Jo with her media assignment

MY CHILD'S TARGET ACTIVITY THIS WEEK:

Activity:

Day/time they can do this activity:

Where they can do this activity:

Anything that might get in the way:

How they can make sure it happens:

What I can do to help and support them:

Before next time we would ask your child to:
Fill in the activity log over the week
Look through and edit their values worksheet. We will review these next session to see how they got on
Try one small valued activity this week.

Brief BA Session 4 Checklist

ID/Client initials:

Date:

Brief BA Session 4 Checklist ***Young person seen alone for majority of the session***	
Complete?	**Task**
	Audio/video recorder on
	Anything in particular to make time for today? Details:
	Complete ROMs: • Young person symptom questionnaire (e.g. RCADS Depression Subscale + Risk Q, or full RCADS if not done recently) • Young person functioning/quality of life questionnaire (e.g. ORS) • Parent report of young person symptom questionnaire (e.g. RCADS Depression Subscale + Risk Q, or full RCADS if not done recently) • Parent report of young person functioning/quality of life questionnaire (e.g. ORS)
	Risk discussion
	Review goal progress (if appropriate)
	Bridge from last time (suggestions of points raised last time to revisit):
	Review activity monitoring
	Review values worksheet
	Valued activities worksheet
	Agree homework: complete activity log, complete valued activities worksheet
	Photocopy young person's completed session worksheets
	Give young person session worksheets to take away
	Give parent session worksheets to take away
	Confirm next session date, time, location
	Young person session feedback questionnaire (e.g. SRS)

After Session 4	
Complete?	**Task**
	Upload audio/video recording and delete from device
	Score young person and parent ROMs (if not done in session)
	Outcome electronic diary appointment (if applicable)
	Electronic or paper session record: ROMs, risk, attendees, content, homework, next appointment
	Upload completed session worksheets and ROMs to electronic records (if applicable)
	Diary appointment for next session
	Prepare to discuss in supervision
	Book room for next session

Young Person Brief BA Session 4 Worksheet

We talked about life areas and values last session, and how important it is to get a *balance* of activities across different life areas.

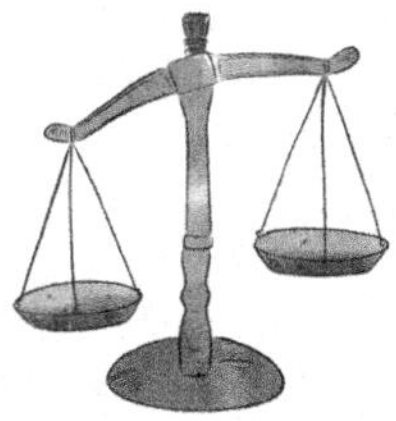

Remember, values are like a compass showing you the direction you want to go in, rather than a destination you can say you've got to – valued activities are a way of moving in the right direction.

LAVA (Life Areas, Values and Activities)

The LAVA worksheets are used to help identify activities that fit with your personal values. You can also rate the activity based on how important and enjoyable you think the activity will be (using a 0–10 scale). You can write as many down as you can think of, as there's no limit.

Break big activities into smaller steps.

Activities can be broken into small steps. For example, if your valued activity is 'Going for a bike ride', there are a number of steps before you can do this. These include getting your bike out of the garage, checking the air in the tyres, finding a tyre pump, pumping the tyres, getting your bike helmet, etc. So the first step in the activity 'Going for a bike ride' might be checking that the bike is in good shape (tyres, lights etc.), deciding where to cycle to, and later going on the actual ride. Activities are much easier to do if they are broken into the smallest pieces possible.

Choose activities that you can do.

We want you to succeed. To improve the chance of success it's a good idea to start with activities that are easier, or that you are doing already but would like to do more often or for longer (see your activity log for ideas).

LAVA tips:

- Try to think about more than one area of your life so you get a spread of reward
- Try to include *Enjoyable* and *Important* activities on your LAVA worksheet – ideally some that are high on both!
- No activity is too small. It's better to think about smaller, achievable tasks that you can realistically do than huge tasks that are easy to put off or may be tricky to do in practice
- It's useful to think about activities that aren't on your activity log, but would have been before you got depressed, or new activities you have always wanted to try
- Remember that activities should relate to your values, as this makes sure they are things you really want to do
- Going back to your activity log, are there some life areas where you have very few activities? This type of information can help us with activity selection and planning.

LAVA example: Sofia

Life area: Me				
Value: Keep active		**Enjoyment (0–10)**	**Importance (0–10)**	**How easy? (0–10)**
Activity 1	Get off the bus a stop early each day	3	4	6
Activity 2	Walk the dog twice at the weekend	7	8	7
Activity 3	Do exercise DVD at home once a week	6	7	4

Life area: Things that matter				
Value: Be organized		**Enjoyment (0–10)**	**Importance (0–10)**	**How easy? (0–10)**
Activity 1	Tidy my room on Sunday evening	4	6	3
Activity 2	Pack my bag the night before school	2	8	9
Activity 3	Plan Saturday's meet up with Carly the day before	8	7	8

Life area: People who matter				
Value: Be a caring friend		**Enjoyment (0–10)**	**Importance (0–10)**	**How easy? (0–10)**
Activity 1	Save a seat for Gina on the bus	7	7	9
Activity 2	Write Tom an email	6	8	6
Activity 3	Ask one friend a day how they are doing	4	7	5

LAVA example: Jayden

Life area: Me				
Value: Get involved in team sports		**Enjoyment (0–10)**	**Importance (0–10)**	**How easy? (0–10)**
Activity 1	Text David to find out when the basketball team train	3	5	9
Activity 2	Go to watch the Sunday football match at the park	8	7	2
Activity 3	Invite Jo round to watch the rugby	7	6	5

Life area: Things that matter				
Value: Improve my career prospects		**Enjoyment (0–10)**	**Importance (0–10)**	**How easy? (0–10)**
Activity 1	Go to my Saturday job to get more experience	3	8	4
Activity 2	Look online at part-time courses	4	6	7
Activity 3	Go to the Careers Advice Service at college	4	7	5

Life area: People who matter				
Value: Help Dad out		**Enjoyment (0–10)**	**Importance (0–10)**	**How easy? (0–10)**
Activity 1	Hoover once a week	2	7	3
Activity 2	Pick up food for dinner on Wednesdays	5	6	7
Activity 3	Go to visit my grandparents when Dad is at work	7	8	8

My LAVA worksheet

Life area: Me (hobbies/fun, physical health, looking after myself)				
Value:		**Enjoyment (0–10)**	**Importance (0–10)**	**How easy? (0–10)**
Activity 1				
Activity 2				
Activity 3				

Life area: Things that matter (education/work, things I need to do, the bigger picture)				
Value:		**Enjoyment (0–10)**	**Importance (0–10)**	**How easy? (0–10)**
Activity 1				
Activity 2				
Activity 3				

Life area: People who matter (family, friends, important other(s))				
Value:		**Enjoyment (0–10)**	**Importance (0–10)**	**How easy? (0–10)**
Activity 1				
Activity 2				
Activity 3				

Before next time:

Have another look at your values worksheet and make sure we've got it right with your values for the different life areas

Continue completing the LAVA worksheets

Plan in three small valued activities – we will review how these went next time.

TARGET ACTIVITIES:

Activity 1:

Day/time I can do this activity:

Activity 2:

Day/time I can do this activity:

Activity 3:

Day/time I can do this activity:

Notes from today's session:

Parent Brief BA Session 4 Worksheet

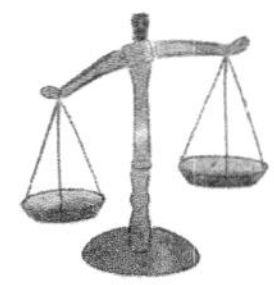

We introduced life areas and values last session, and discussed how important it is to get a balance of activities across different life areas. This applies to all of us, but particularly for people who are experiencing depression, as they tend to have lost that 'feel-good' factor from life that values can bring.

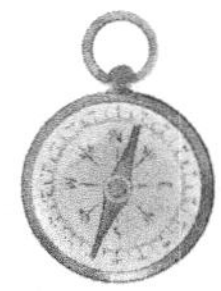

The life areas and values worksheet can help us understand your child's values. Remember, values are like a compass showing your child the direction they want to go in, rather than a destination they actually get to – valued activities are a way of moving in the right direction.

Life areas recap

Me	Things that matter	People who matter
Hobbies/fun	Education or work	Family
Physical health	Everyday stuff	Friends
Looking after myself	The bigger picture	Important other(s)

Valued activities recap

Valued activities are things your child can do to live according to their values. They are useful to think about because:

- Without activities that help your child live according to their values, values are just words and ideas, not a reality
- Activities are things your child actually can *do* as opposed to something your child thinks or feels, so are *easier to monitor and plan*
- There can be more than one activity your child can do to fit with a value, which gives us more chance to come up with a variety of activities they can plan into their week and more options to draw on if one of these isn't possible.

Activities are specific ways for your child to head in the direction of their values.

LAVA (Life Areas, Values and Activities)

The LAVA worksheets at the end of this session allow your child to identify their values across key areas of their life. For each life area, your child has space for both values and activities. Each activity should be something that your child can do to live consistently with the value that they identified. There are some example worksheets already completed by Sofia and Jayden to show them how to do this.

When planning the activity, your child will also rate the activity based on how important or enjoyable they think the activity will be (*using a 0–10 scale*). This will be useful later to compare how important or enjoyable the activity actually is when your child does it.

Break big activities into smaller steps.

It's important to help your child succeed when they try out valued activities. Therefore activities should be broken into smaller parts. For example, if the valued activity is 'Going for a bike ride', a number of intermediate steps are required before your child can do this. These might include: getting the bike out of the garage, checking the air in the tyres, finding a tyre pump, finding their bike helmet and lights, pumping the tyres, etc. So the first step in the activity of 'Going for a bike ride' might be 'Check that the bike is in good shape', the next step could be 'Collect lights, helmet and pump'. The next step could be 'Go for a bike ride'. Activities are far easier to achieve if they are broken into the smallest pieces possible.

Help your child choose activities they can do.

It is also important to select activities from very simple to more difficult. To improve the likelihood of initial success, some of the activities your child chooses should be ones they are already doing regularly but would like to do more often or for longer (your child's activity log may provide some ideas). Your child's therapist will review their values and activity log in the session and help them identify valued activities. They can continue to add to their activity log and edit it on their own, or with your help.

By expanding your child's valued activities to cover different aspects of their life, you can maximize their opportunity to have positive experiences.

LAVA tips:

- It is important for your child to identify values in more than one area of their life so they are looking at getting reward from different areas. This helps spread the chance of getting reward from life – a bit like the saying 'Don't put all your eggs in one basket'
- It helps if your child has *both Enjoyable and Important* activities on their LAVA worksheet – ideally some that are high on both!
- No activity is too small. It's better to think about smaller, achievable tasks that your child can realistically do than huge tasks that are easy to put off or may be tricky to do in practice
- It's good to think about activities that aren't on your child's activity log at the moment, but would have been before your child got depressed, or new activities your child has always wanted to try. You can help by encouraging them to consider small, achievable activities and offering your support to help make these happen
- One of the most important things is recognizing your child's values, as that makes it much easier to see where the gaps are (i.e. values your child might want to pay more attention to by doing activities linked to these)
- Going back to your child's activity log, are there some life areas where your child has very few activities? This type of information can help with selecting and planning activities

- Keep in mind how difficult your child might find doing some activities, even if they are things they used to do very easily or previously enjoyed. It will take more effort to overcome depression symptoms and get going, so any way you can encourage them or show them you recognize their effort will be helpful.

Before next time we would ask your child to:

Have another look at their values worksheet and make sure we've got it right with their values for the different life areas

Continue completing the LAVA worksheets

Plan in three small valued activities – we will review how these went next time.

TARGET ACTIVITIES:

Three activities my child thinks they will be able to do, when, and how I can help:

Activity 1:

Day/time they can do this activity:

I can help by:

Activity 2:

Day/time they can do this activity:

I can help by:

Activity 3:

Day/time they can do this activity:

I can help by:

LAVA example: Sofia

Life area: Me				
Value: Keep active		**Enjoyment (0–10)**	**Importance (0–10)**	**How easy? (0–10)**
Activity 1	Get off the bus a stop early each day	3	4	6
Activity 2	Walk the dog twice at the weekend	7	8	7
Activity 3	Do exercise DVD at home once a week	6	7	4

Life area: Things that matter				
Value: Be organized		**Enjoyment (0–10)**	**Importance (0–10)**	**How easy? (0–10)**
Activity 1	Tidy my room on Sunday evening	4	6	3
Activity 2	Pack my bag the night before school	2	8	9
Activity 3	Plan Saturday's meet up with Carly the day before	8	7	8

Life area: People who matter				
Value: Be a caring friend		**Enjoyment (0–10)**	**Importance (0–10)**	**How easy? (0–10)**
Activity 1	Save a seat for Gina on the bus	7	7	9
Activity 2	Write Tom an email	6	8	6
Activity 3	Ask one friend a day how they are doing	4	7	5

LAVA example: Jayden

Life area: Me				
Value: Get involved in team sports		**Enjoyment (0–10)**	**Importance (0–10)**	**How easy? (0–10)**
Activity 1	Text David to find out when the basketball team train	3	5	9
Activity 2	Go to watch the Sunday football match at the park	8	7	2
Activity 3	Invite Jo round to watch the rugby	7	6	5

Life area: Things that matter				
Value: Improve my career prospects		**Enjoyment (0–10)**	**Importance (0–10)**	**How easy? (0–10)**
Activity 1	Go to my Saturday job to get more experience	3	8	4
Activity 2	Look online at part-time courses	4	6	7
Activity 3	Go to the Careers Advice Service at college	4	7	5

Life area: People who matter				
Value: Help Dad out		**Enjoyment (0–10)**	**Importance (0–10)**	**How easy? (0–10)**
Activity 1	Hoover once a week	2	7	3
Activity 2	Pick up food for dinner on Wednesdays	5	6	7
Activity 3	Go to visit my grandparents when Dad is at work	7	8	8

My LAVA worksheet

Life area: Me (hobbies/fun, physical health, looking after myself)				
Value:		**Enjoyment (0–10)**	**Importance (0–10)**	**How easy? (0–10)**
Activity 1				
Activity 2				
Activity 3				

Life area: Things that matter (education/work, things I need to do, the bigger picture)				
Value:		**Enjoyment (0–10)**	**Importance (0–10)**	**How easy? (0–10)**
Activity 1				
Activity 2				
Activity 3				

Life area: People who matter (family, friends, important other(s))				
Value:		**Enjoyment (0–10)**	**Importance (0–10)**	**How easy? (0–10)**
Activity 1				
Activity 2				
Activity 3				

Brief BA Session 5 Checklist

ID/Client initials:

Date:

Brief BA Session 5 Checklist *Young person seen alone for majority of the session*	
Complete?	**Task**
	Audio/video recorder on
	Anything in particular to make time for today? Details:
	Complete ROMs: • Young person symptom questionnaire (e.g. RCADS Depression Subscale + Risk Q, or full RCADS if not done recently) • Young person functioning/quality of life questionnaire (e.g. ORS) • Parent report of young person symptom questionnaire (e.g. RCADS Depression Subscale + Risk Q, or full RCADS if not done recently) • Parent report of young person functioning/quality of life questionnaire (e.g. ORS)
	Risk discussion
	Review goal progress if appropriate
	Bridge from last time (suggestions of points raised last time to revisit):
	Review activity monitoring (including troubleshooting if not completed valued activities)
	Review values worksheet and LAVA worksheet
	Identify activities: • Currently doing • Want to do • Need help with
	Agree homework: complete activity log, try out activities you've planned
	Photocopy young person's completed session worksheets
	Give young person session worksheets to take away
	Give parent session worksheets to take away
	Confirm next session date, time, location
	Young person session feedback questionnaire (e.g. SRS)

After session 5	
Complete?	**Task**
	Upload audio/video recording and delete from device
	Score young person and parent ROMs (if not done in session)
	Outcome electronic diary appointment (if applicable)
	Electronic or paper session record: ROMs, risk, attendees, content, homework, next appointment
	Upload completed session worksheets and ROMs to electronic records (if applicable)
	Diary appointment for next session
	Prepare to discuss in supervision
	Book room for next session

Young Person Brief BA Session 5 Worksheet

Selecting valued activities

The activities you choose should be easy to measure and observe, and directly related to the values you listed on the values worksheet.

The more the activities are linked to your values, the more likely it is that they will be meaningful for you.

Finding a balance

It's important that you have a balance of activities across different life areas. If you only ever did activities that were about getting good grades at school, there would be a lot of other areas of your life that wouldn't be getting enough attention. This can keep depression going, as there aren't many opportunities to feel close to others and enjoy yourself while doing schoolwork, even if you feel it's important and you're achieving something. Equally, if you never felt you were doing anything that gave you a sense of achievement, that wouldn't be a good balance either.

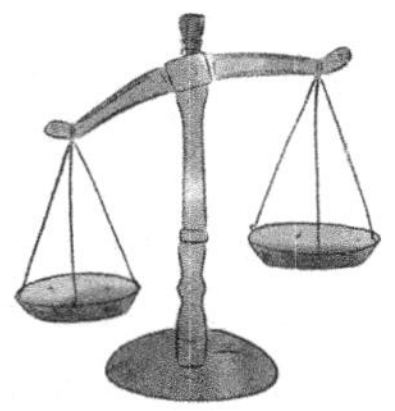

The balance across life areas is important.

Activity example: Sofia

Activities Sofia is doing: Sofia's activity log shows she spends lots of her time on activities related to the 'Things that matter' value of doing well at school. She feels pressure from her parents to keep up with activities like her piano lessons that don't fit with any of her values and she doesn't really enjoy any more.

Activities Sofia would like to do: Sofia would like to do more activities focused on the 'Me' and 'People who matter' life areas:

Have a film night with Andy

Walk the dog

Have a pamper evening with Carly

Join a group exercise class

Help out at the animal shelter

Speak to at least one person in every lesson

Go to church on Sundays with Mum

Help Dad wash the car

Activities Sofia needs help to do: Sofia needs help from her parents to agree she should stop her piano lessons, and to give her the money to go to the exercise class. She'd like her friend Emma to join with her.

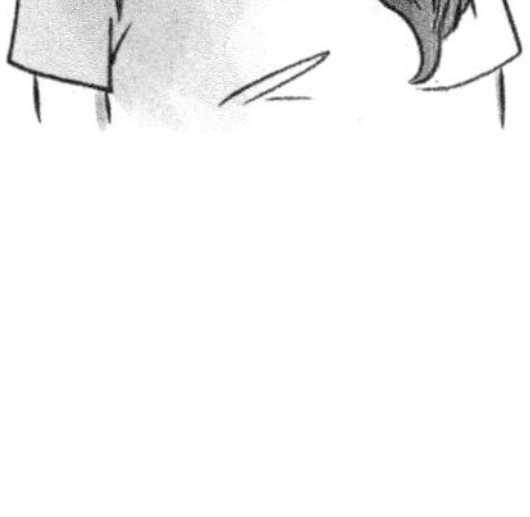

Activity example: Jayden

Activities Jayden is doing: Jayden has noticed that his activity log has very few entries that are important to him, and his ACE levels are pretty low across the board.

Activities Jayden would like to do: Jayden would like to add in activities that relate to his values in all three life areas: 'Me', 'Things that matter' and 'People who matter':

Re-join the basketball team

Clear up my bedroom

Help Dad cook dinner

Go to my Saturday job at the garden centre

Get up before 10am during the week

Visit my grandparents

Spend 15 minutes sorting out the garden

Help out at the community centre

Go to Jamie's house to hang out with him

Activities Jayden needs help to do: Jayden isn't sure when the basketball team trains anymore, so he needs to find out. He knows he will have to speak to the Community Centre Manager about volunteering. He also thinks he might need some help from his dad to get out of bed earlier each day.

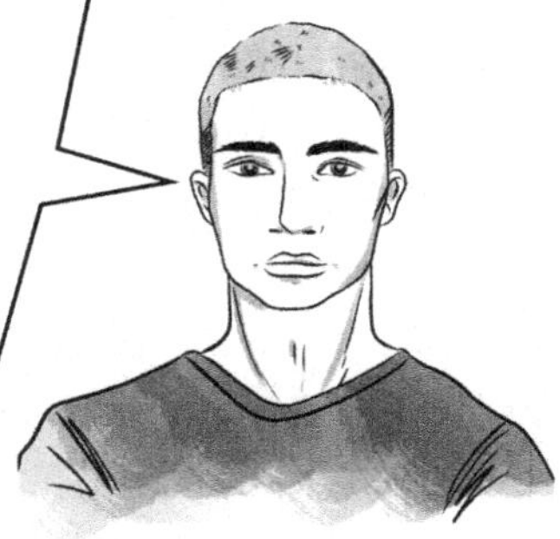

Target activities

We want to have a list of target activities you *really* want to try, and then plan how you're going to try them out.

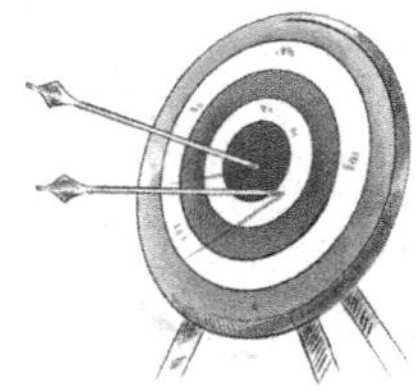

Remember, it's your choice which activities to target.

Making activities achievable

- Make sure you pick activities you are ready to try
- If there are barriers to doing an activity, we can discuss ways to overcome these
- Make sure you have broken activities down into their smallest parts, for example going to the gym might involve these smaller activities:
  - Get gym clothes
  - Find a gym
  - Arrange a lift to and from the gym
  - Find a friend who wants to go too.

Why do I have to plan exactly when I will do the activity?

By planning a day and time, and writing this down, it makes it much more likely that you won't forget. It can be easy to *not* try them, but writing them down and being specific gives you a goal to aim for.

Thinking about a specific day and time you will do each activity will make you really think through where you can realistically fit the activity into your schedule and make it more likely you will do it.

How will this help me feel better?

When you begin to complete the activities, you will be acting in a way that fits with what matters to *you*, your values in different life areas. You might not feel any better straightaway, but over time you will be breaking the vicious cycle of depression and having many more opportunities for getting more of the 'feel-good' factor in your life.

Activities I do already that fit with my values:

Activities I want to do that fit with my values:

Activities that fit with my values but I need help to do:

Parent Brief BA Session 5 Worksheet

Selecting valued activities

By now your child should be starting to have an idea of what valued activities might be possible to add into their every-day life. The activities your child chooses should be easy to measure and observe, and directly related to their personal values. The more the activities are linked to your child's values, the more likely it is that the activities will be meaningful for them and therefore be easier to try out, and more rewarding to do.

Finding a balance

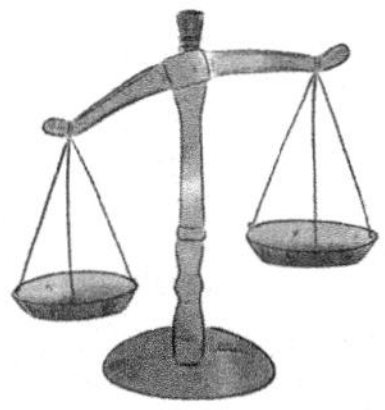

It's important that your child has a balance of activities that relate to different life areas. If your child only ever did activities that were about getting good grades at school, there would be a lot of other areas of their life that would not get enough attention. This can keep depression going, as there aren't many opportunities for your child to feel close to others and enjoy themselves while doing schoolwork, even if your child feels it's important and that they are achieving something. Equally, if they weren't doing anything that gave them a sense of achievement, this would not be a good balance either. While there may be times in life that the balance is a little focused on one area more than others (e.g. during exam time), it's important that even during these periods your child plans in activities that fit with values across other parts of their life.

The balance across life areas, as well as the number of activities, is important.

Activity example: Sofia

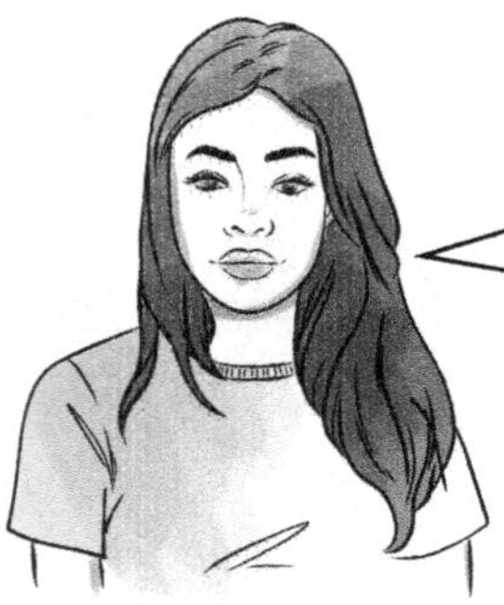

Activities Sofia is doing: Sofia's activity log shows that she spends lots of her time on activities related to the 'Things that matter' value of doing well at school. She feels pressure from her parents to keep up with activities like her piano lessons that don't fit with any of her values and she doesn't really enjoy any more.

Activities Sofia would like to do: Sofia would like to do more activities focused on the 'Me' and 'People who matter' life areas:

- Have a film night with Andy
- Walk the dog
- Have a pamper evening with Carly
- Join a group exercise class
- Help out at the animal shelter
- Speak to at least one person in every lesson
- Go to church on Sundays with Mum
- Help Dad wash the car

Activities Sofia needs help to do: Sofia needs help from her parents to agree she should stop her piano lessons, and to give her the money to go to the exercise class. She'd like her friend Emma to join her.

Activity example: Jayden

Activities Jayden is doing: Jayden has noticed that his activity log has very few entries that are important to him, and his ACE levels are pretty low across the board.

Activities Jayden would like to do: Jayden would like to add in activities that relate to his values in all three life areas: 'Me', 'Things that matter' and 'People who matter':

Re-join the basketball team

Clear up my bedroom

Help Dad cook dinner

Go to my Saturday job at the garden centre

Get up before 10am during the week

Visit my grandparents

Spend 15 minutes sorting out the garden

Help out at the community centre

Go to Jamie's house to hang out with him

Activities Jayden needs help to do: Jayden isn't sure when the basketball team trains any more, so he needs to find out. He knows he will have to speak to the Community Centre Manager about volunteering. He also thinks he might need some help from his dad to get out of bed earlier each day.

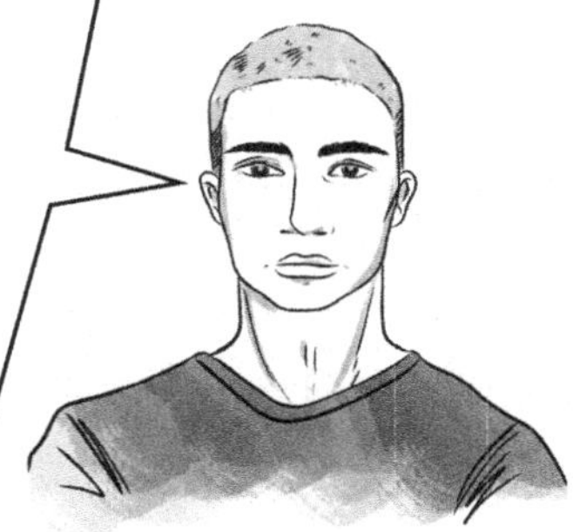

Target activities

We want to have a list of target activities your child *really* wants to try. Once your child is happy with their target activities, we need to plan how they are going to try them out and review progress.

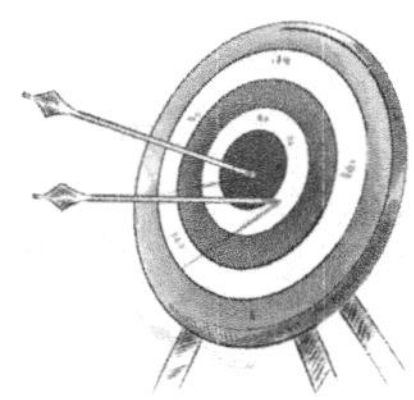

Remember, it's your child's choice which activities to target, but you can help them come up with ideas and encourage them with this.

Making activities achievable

- It's important your child picks activities they are ready to try
- If there are barriers to doing an activity, can you help your child overcome these?
- Make sure your child has broken activities down into their smallest parts, for example going to the gym might involve these smaller activities:
  - Get gym clothes
  - Find a gym
  - Arrange a lift to and from the gym
  - Find a friend or family member to join them

- At this stage, it's helpful to encourage even small efforts towards positive behaviour, and completing smaller steps towards a bigger activity is much easier than aiming for the larger task all in one go.

Why does my child have to plan exactly when they will do the activity?

By planning a day and time, and writing this down, it makes it much more likely that your child won't forget to do the activity. We all know this from our own experience. It can also be easy to not try new activities (due to the symptoms of depression actively fighting against this), but writing them down and being specific gives your child a goal to aim for.

Thinking about a specific day and time when your child will do each activity will make them really think through where they can realistically fit the activity into their schedule. This makes it more likely that your child will do it. You can also help with this – knowing when and where they plan to do the activity means that you can help support them doing this (e.g. by reminding them, encouraging them, offering a lift or company to do an activity).

How will this help my child feel better?

When your child begins to complete valued activities, they will be acting in a way that fits with what matters to them, with their values in different life areas. Your child might not feel better straightaway (and it's important to remember that this is unlikely), but over time they will break the vicious cycle of depression and have many more opportunities for getting positive reinforcement and reward in their life.

Activities my child does already:

Activities my child wants to do:

Activities my child needs help to do:

Brief BA Session 6 Checklist

ID/Client initials:

Date:

Brief BA Session 6 Checklist *Agree with family how to split session: some time with young person and parent but also time with young person alone*	
Complete?	**Task**
	Audio/video recorder on
	Anything in particular to make time for today? Details:
	Complete ROMs: • Young person symptom questionnaire (e.g. RCADS Depression Subscale + Risk Q, or full RCADS if not done recently) • Young person functioning/quality of life questionnaire (e.g. ORS) • Parent report of young person symptom questionnaire (e.g. RCADS Depression Subscale + Risk Q, or full RCADS if not done recently) • Parent report of young person functioning/quality of life questionnaire (e.g. ORS)
	Risk discussion
	Review goal progress if appropriate
	Bridge from last time (suggestions of points raised last time to revisit):
	Review activity monitoring and scheduling
	Plan future activities
	Contracts
	Problem-solving
	Agree homework: complete activity log, try out activities you've planned, use contracts or problem-solving if required
	Photocopy young person's completed session worksheets
	Give young person session worksheets to take away
	Give parent session worksheets to take away
	Confirm next session date, time, location
	Young person session feedback questionnaire (e.g. SRS)
	Parent session feedback questionnaire (e.g. SRS)

After Session 6	
Complete?	**Task**
	Upload audio/video recording and delete from device
	Score young person and parent ROMs (if not done in session)
	Outcome electronic diary appointment (if applicable)
	Electronic or paper session record: ROMs, risk, attendees, content, homework, next appointment
	Upload completed session worksheets and ROMs to electronic records (if applicable)
	Diary appointment for next session
	Prepare to discuss in supervision
	Book room for next session

Young Person Brief BA Session 6 Worksheet

Progress review

How are things now? What's changed since we first met?

How would you explain Brief BA to someone in three sentences?

Contracts

Sometimes we need help completing our activities. It might be that we need a lift to the cinema to watch a film with our friends, a hand getting some sports equipment from the loft, or help from a teacher to finish a tricky piece of coursework.

This is where contracts can come in useful. Just as we need to be specific with the activities we are doing, it also helps to be specific with what help we are going to need and who might be able to help us with it.

Contracts example: Sofia

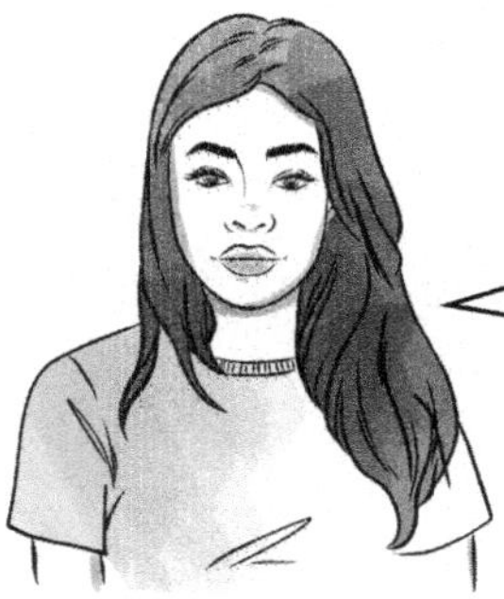

Sofia decides that she wants to go to her friend Emma's house to watch a film on Wednesday night. Emma lives a 10-minute drive away or a 20-minute bus ride away from Sofia's house. Sofia uses a contract with her dad so she can get to her friend's house.

Activity: **I need to get to and from Emma's house for a film night**

Name one person who can help you with this activity: **Dad**

What are the ways this person can help you with this activity?

1) Dad could give me a lift to Emma's house

2) I could borrow some money from Dad to catch the bus to Emma's house

Contracts example: Jayden

Jayden wants to help out at the community centre; he has been told that he needs to complete an application form for this but he is unsure of how to go about it. Jayden uses a contract to get the help he needs.

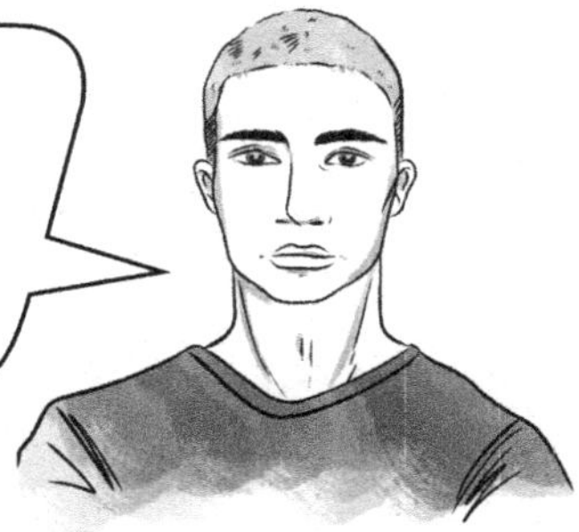

Activity: **Fill out an application form for the community centre**

Name one person who can help you with this activity: **John Taylor (Community Centre Manager)**

What are the ways this person can help you with this activity?

1) Ask John for some time to go through the application form together

2) Email John for some advice on what to include

Your contracts

Together, what is an activity you could use some help to complete?

Activity (when, where):

Name one person who can help you with this activity:

What are the ways this person can help you with this activity?

Problem-solving

When you are trying to make changes in your life, things can get in the way and make it difficult. We don't want this to stop you, so a useful way to troubleshoot problems is shown in the steps below:

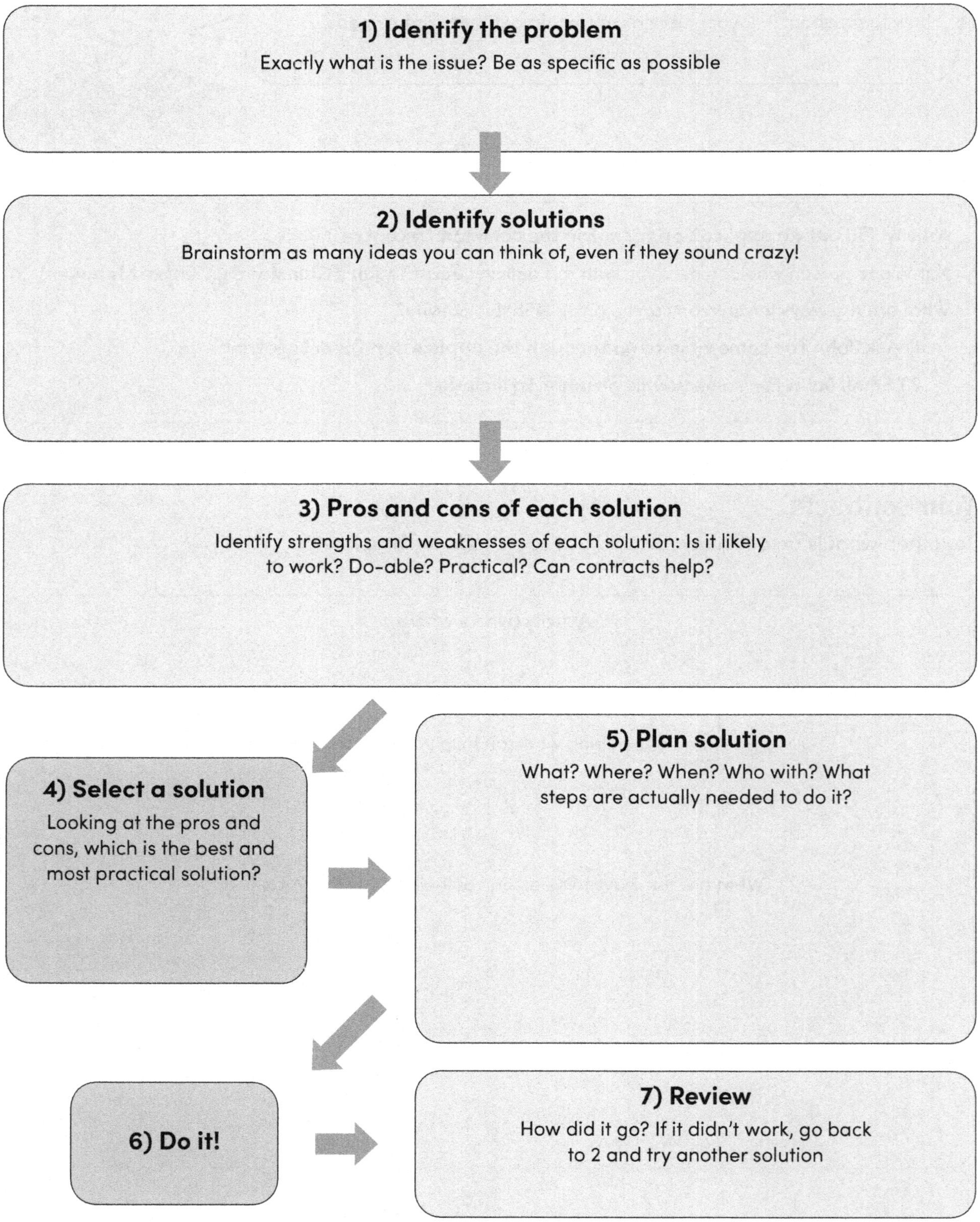

PROBLEM-SOLVING FLOWCHART

Before next time:

Keep doing more of what matters to you, by planning in and doing valued activities across different life areas

Over the next week, complete the activity log but highlight each planned activity on the log if you completed it (and fill in the ratings too)

Try using contracts and/or problem-solving to stop things getting in the way of progress

We will review this together next time we meet to see how you got on.

Notes from today's session:

Parent Brief BA Session 6 Worksheet

Progress review

How are things now? What's changed for your child since we first met?

How would you explain Brief BA to someone in three sentences?

Contracts

Sometimes we need help completing activities, and we could all benefit from a bit of practical help with certain things. You will know from your own experience that some tasks are much easier when you have the support of someone else, especially if they are able to make it easier, or are the ones who can make the activity happen. Children and young people often need some support from adults to do certain activities, and this is normal. It might be that they need a lift to the cinema to watch a film with their friends, a hand getting some sports equipment from the loft, or they may need some help from a teacher to finish a tricky piece of coursework. When a young person is depressed, they may need extra help to make valued activities possible (especially when they are fighting against depression symptoms that get in the way of doing these things).

This is where contracts can come in useful. Just as we need to be specific in specifying the valued activities we are doing, it also helps to be specific with what help we are going to need and who might be able to help us with it.

Contracts example: Sofia

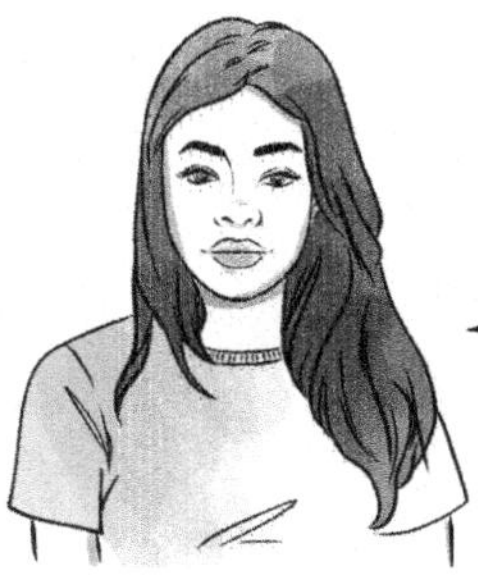

Sofia decides that she wants to go to her friend Emma's house to watch a film on Wednesday night. Emma lives a 10-minute drive away or a 20-minute bus ride away from Sofia's house. Sofia uses a contract with her dad so she can get to her friend's house.

Activity: **I need to get to and from Emma's house for a film night**

Name one person who can help you with this activity: **Dad**

What are the ways this person can help you with this activity?

1) Dad could give me a lift to Emma's house

2) I could borrow some money from Dad to catch the bus to Emma's house

Contracts example: Jayden

Jayden wants to help out at the community centre; he has been told that he needs to complete an application form for this but he is unsure of how to go about it. Jayden uses a contract to get the help he needs.

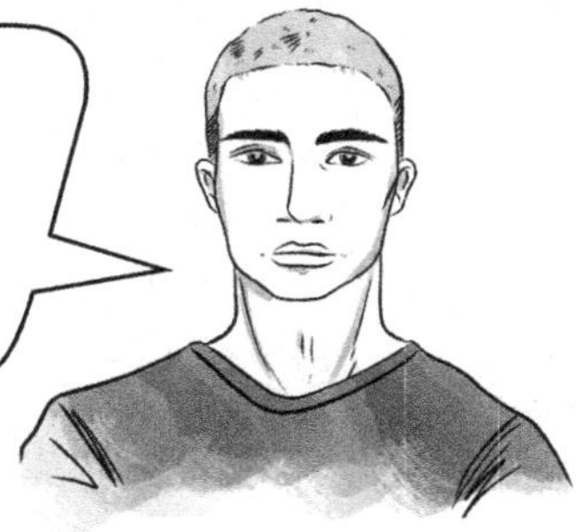

Activity: **Fill out an application form for the community centre**

Name one person who can help your child with this activity: **John Taylor (Community Centre Manager)**

What are the ways this person can help you with this activity?

1) Ask John for some time to go through the application form together

2) Email John for some advice on what to include

Your child's contracts

What valued activity could your child use some help to complete?

Activity (when, where):

Name one person who can help you with this activity:

What are the ways this person can help you with this activity?

Problem-solving

When your child is trying to make changes in their life, things can get in the way and make it difficult. We don't want these to stop your child, so a useful way to troubleshoot problems is shown in the steps below. This is a method you may already know about and use in your everyday life (many adults use problem-solving as a key part of their jobs or roles). However, this isn't a technique young people are formally taught, and the brain areas that help you problem-solve are still developing in adolescents. This is why we have included this practical flowchart. It can be used for any kind of problem-solving your child may need some help with, and can be a good tool to use together if they are struggling with something.

1) Identify the problem

Exactly what is the issue? Be as specific as possible

2) Identify solutions

Brainstorm as many ideas you can think of, even if they sound crazy!

3) Pros and cons of each solution

Identify strengths and weaknesses of each solution: Is it likely to work? Do-able? Practical? Can contracts help?

4) Select a solution

Looking at the pros and cons, which is the best and most practical solution?

5) Plan solution

What? Where? When? Who with? What steps are actually needed to do it?

6) Do it!

7) Review

How did it go? If it didn't work, go back to 2 and try another solution

PROBLEM-SOLVING FLOWCHART

Before next time we would ask your child to:

Keep doing more of what matters to them, by planning and doing valued activities

Over the next week, complete their activity log but highlight each planned activity on their log if they completed it (and fill in the ratings too)

Try using contracts and/or problem-solving to stop things getting in the way of progress

We will review this together next time we meet to see how your child got on.

Notes from today's session:

Brief BA Session 7 Checklist

ID/Client initials:

Date:

Brief BA Session 7 Checklist ***Young person seen alone for majority of the session***	
Complete?	**Task**
	Audio/video recorder on
	Anything in particular to make time for today? Details:
	Complete ROMs: • Young person symptom questionnaire (e.g. RCADS Depression Subscale + Risk Q, or full RCADS if not done recently) • Young person functioning/quality of life questionnaire (e.g. ORS) • Parent report of young person symptom questionnaire (e.g. RCADS Depression Subscale + Risk Q, or full RCADS if not done recently) • Parent report of young person functioning/quality of life questionnaire (e.g. ORS)
	Risk discussion
	Review goal progress if appropriate
	Bridge from last time (suggestions of points raised last time to revisit):
	Review activity monitoring and scheduling
	Recap any other areas as appropriate: • Activity monitoring • Planning in valued activities • Contracts • Problem-solving • Other:
	Identify here and now Brief BA cycle
	Agree homework: complete activity log, try out activities you've planned
	Photocopy young person's completed session worksheets
	Give young person session worksheets to take away
	Give parent session worksheets to take away
	Confirm next session date, time, location
	Young person session feedback questionnaire (e.g. SRS)

After Session 7	
Complete?	**Task**
	Upload audio/video recording and delete from device
	Score young person and parent ROMs (if not done in session)
	Outcome electronic diary appointment (if applicable)
	Electronic or paper session record: ROMs, risk, attendees, content, homework, next appointment
	Upload completed session worksheets and ROMs to electronic records (if applicable)
	Diary appointment for next session
	Prepare to discuss in supervision
	Book room for next session

Young Person Brief BA Session 7 Worksheet

Review of progress: What's changed?

It's helpful to check in about what (if anything) is different now from before starting Brief BA.

Changes example: Jayden

Jayden has filled in his application form for the community centre and is now waiting to hear back about helping out at the youth club. He has managed to get to his Saturday job over the past few weeks, and is now doing the food shopping on the day his dad works a late shift. He still finds it hard to get out of bed every morning, but now tries to plan a visit to his grandparents for lunch twice a week, which means he has a reason to get up.

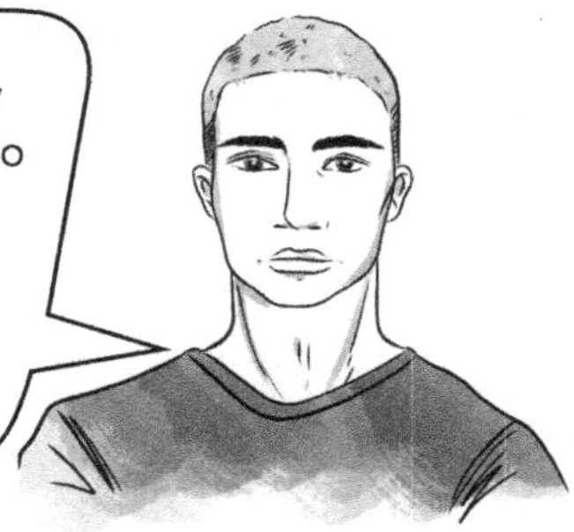

Changes example: Sofia

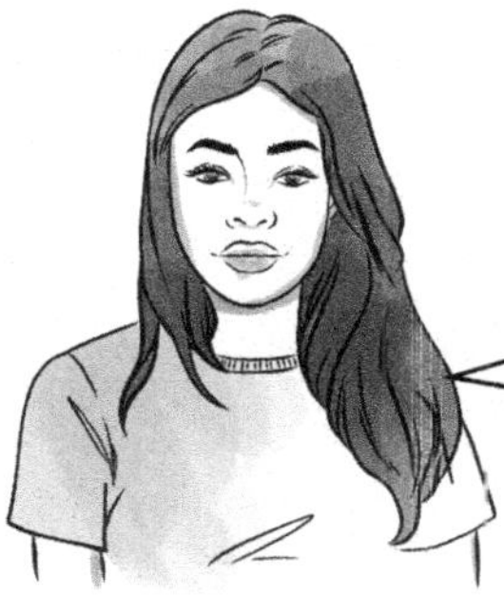

Sofia has agreed with her parents that she will stop her piano lessons, as she wasn't enjoying them anymore. She has also changed her twice-weekly dance class to a drop-in exercise class she goes to with her friend once a fortnight. This has given her more time for herself, where she has time relaxing in the evenings after finishing homework, and she manages to get to bed a bit earlier after reading a book from her favourite series.

What have I changed that's made me feel better?
What do I still want to work on?

Here and now cycle: What are things like for you now?

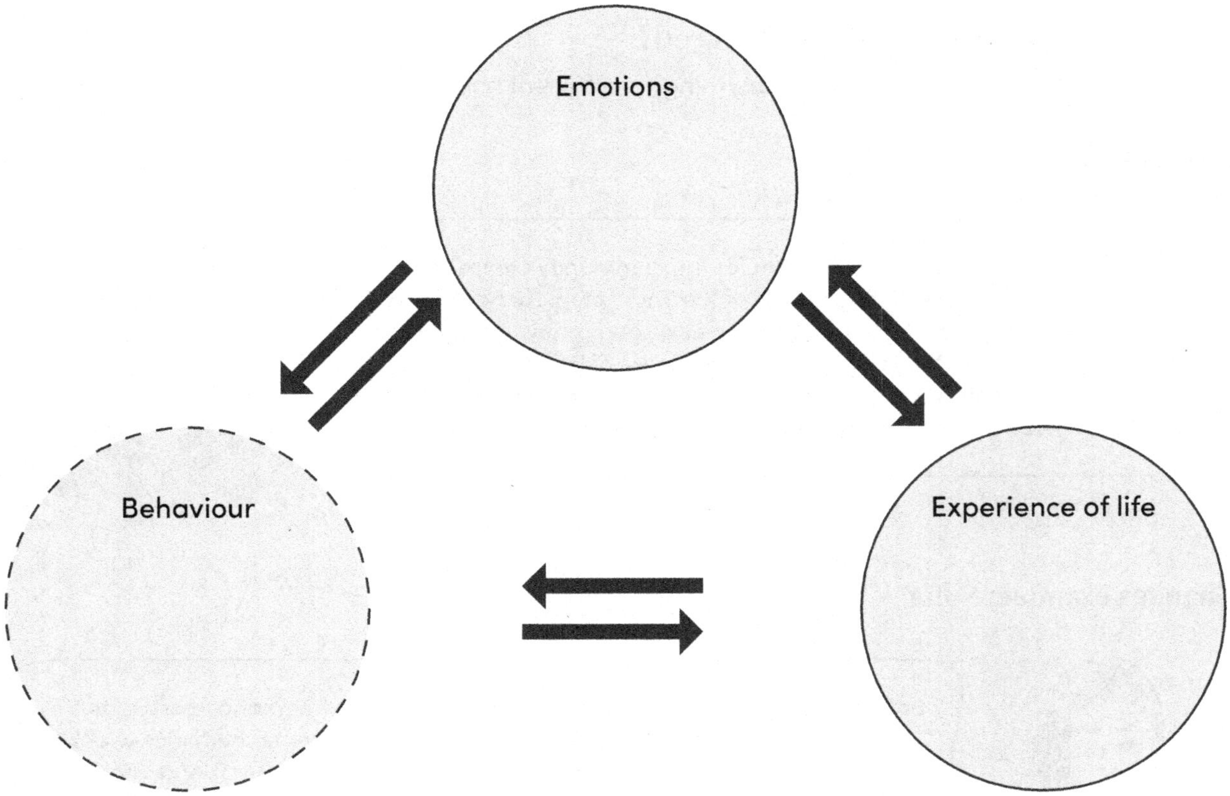

Before next time:

Keep planning and doing valued activities

Fill in your activity log, circling each planned activity on your log if you completed it (and fill in the ratings too)

If you didn't manage to complete the activity, put a line through it and if possible try to re-schedule for later in the week (or even that day)

If you did extra activities deliberately but you didn't plan them in advance, make sure these are added in too!

We will review this together next time we meet to see how you got on.

Parent Brief BA Session 7 Worksheet

Review of progress: What's changed?

It's helpful to check in about what (if anything) is different for your child now compared to before starting Brief BA. Sometimes there aren't many changes but often there is still something positive to identify and encourage.

Changes example: Jayden

Jayden has filled in his application form for the community centre and is now waiting to hear back about helping out at the youth club. He has managed to get to his Saturday job over the past few weeks, and is now doing the food shopping for his dad on a Tuesday. He still finds it hard to get out of bed every morning, but now tries to plan a visit to his grandparents for lunch twice a week, which means he has a reason to get up.

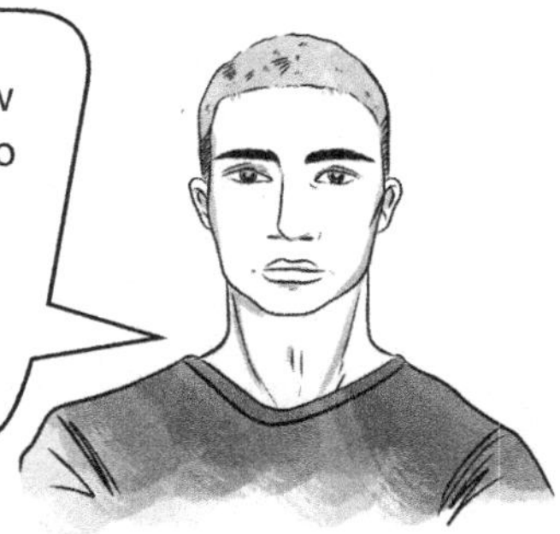

Changes example: Sofia

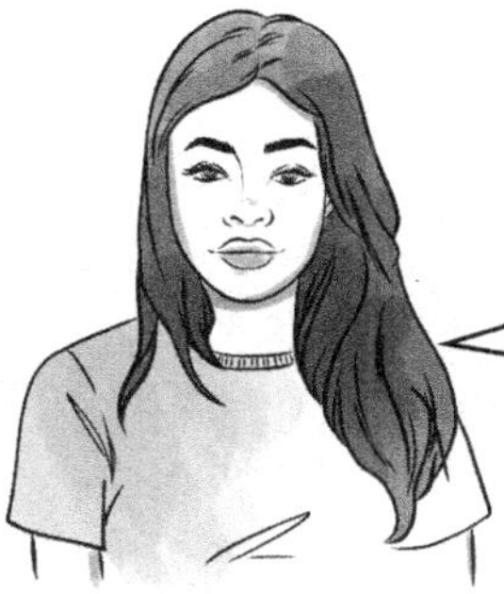

Sofia has agreed with her parents that she will stop her piano lessons, as she wasn't enjoying them anymore. She has also changed her twice-weekly dance class to a drop-in exercise class she goes to with her friend once a fortnight. This has given her more time for herself, where she has time relaxing in the evenings after finishing homework, and she manages to get to bed a bit earlier after reading a book from her favourite series.

What has my child done differently that's helped them feel better?

What do they still want to work on?

How can I help them with this?

Here and now cycle: What are things like for your child now?

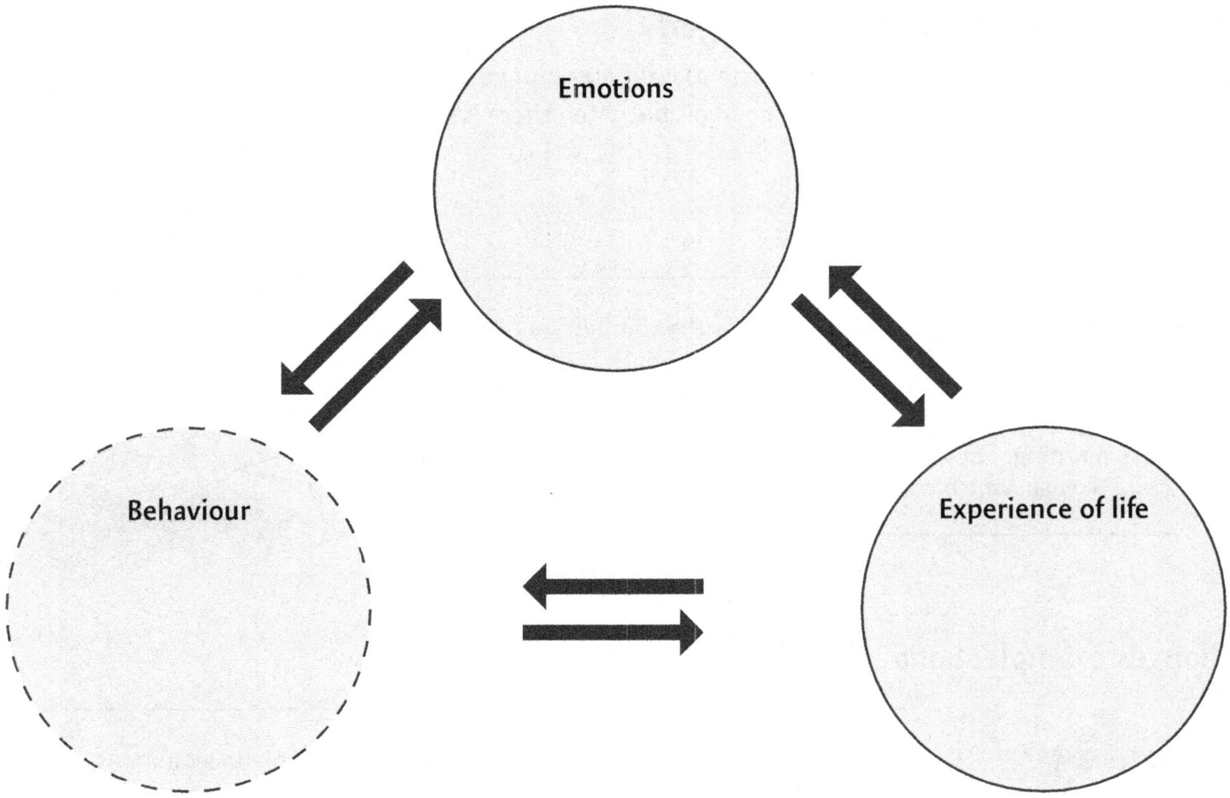

Before next time we would ask your child to:

Keep doing more of what matters to them, by planning and engaging in valued activities

Fill in their activity log, circling each planned activity on the log if they completed it (and fill in the ratings too)

If they didn't manage to complete the activity, put a line through it and if possible try to re-schedule for later in the week (or even that day)

If your child did extra activities deliberately but didn't plan them in advance, make sure these are added in too!

We will review this together next time we meet to see how you got on.

Brief BA Session 8 Checklist

ID/Client initials:

Date:

Brief BA Session 8 Checklist *Agree with family how to split session: some time with young person and parent but also time with young person alone)*	
Complete?	**Task**
	Audio/video recorder on
	Anything in particular to make time for today? Details:
	Complete ROMs: • Young person symptom questionnaire (e.g. RCADS Depression Subscale + Risk Q, or full RCADS if not done recently) • Young person functioning/quality of life questionnaire (e.g. ORS) • Parent report of young person symptom questionnaire (e.g. RCADS Depression Subscale + Risk Q, or full RCADS if not done recently) • Parent report of young person functioning/quality of life questionnaire (e.g. ORS)
	Risk discussion
	Review goal progress if appropriate
	Bridge from last time (suggestions of points raised last time to revisit):
	Recap any other areas as appropriate: • Activity monitoring • Planning in valued activities • Contracts • Problem-solving
	Planning for the future, how to say goodbye next session
	'Healthy Me' worksheet
	Agree homework: continue planning valued activities
	Photocopy young person's completed session worksheets
	Give young person session worksheets to take away
	Give parent session worksheets to take away
	Confirm next session date, time, location
	Young person session feedback questionnaire (e.g. SRS)

After session 8	
Complete?	**Task**
	Upload audio/video recording and delete from device
	Score young person and parent ROMs (if not done in session)
	Outcome electronic diary appointment (if applicable)
	Electronic or paper session record: ROMs, risk, attendees, content, homework, next appointment
	Upload completed session worksheets and ROMs to electronic records (if applicable)
	Diary appointment for next session
	Prepare to discuss in supervision
	Book room for next session

'Healthy Me'

Everyone is different, so it's important to think about what helps *you* stay healthy and happy. Fill in the boxes below and keep this worksheet in a place where you can look at it to remind you in future.

What have I learned about how to keep myself healthy?

What do I need to keep doing, specifically?

What times ahead might be tricky for me?

What are the early warning signs I'm struggling or that my depression symptoms are back?

What can I do when I notice these warning signs?

Who can help me?

Name:

How they can help:

Name:

How they can help:

Name:

How they can help:

Young Person Brief BA Session 8 Worksheet

This session is a recap of the things we've talked about in our Brief BA work, to think about what has been most useful for you and how you can keep using these skills on your own.

Beating depression with Brief BA

1) **Doing** things differently → **LEADS TO** → 2) **Thinking** and **feeling** differently

Activity monitoring

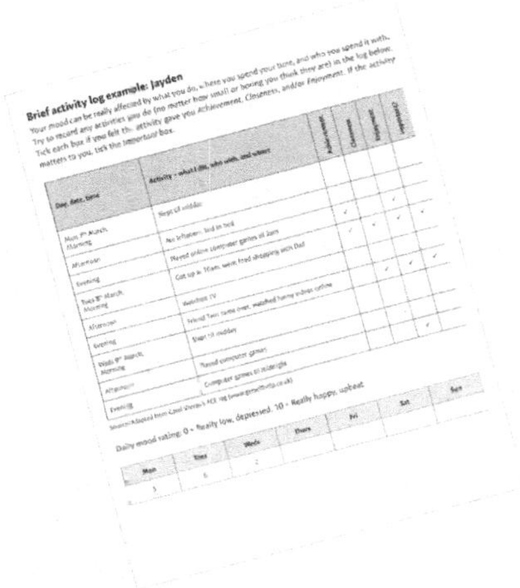
Brief activity log example: Jayden

Activity monitoring

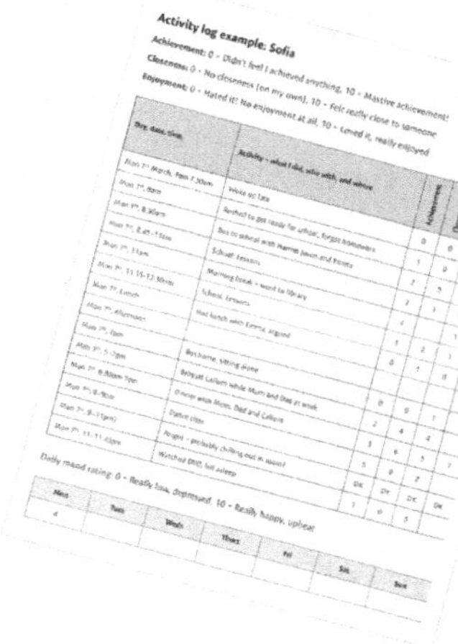
Activity log example: Sofia

Recap: What did I learn by completing my activity log?

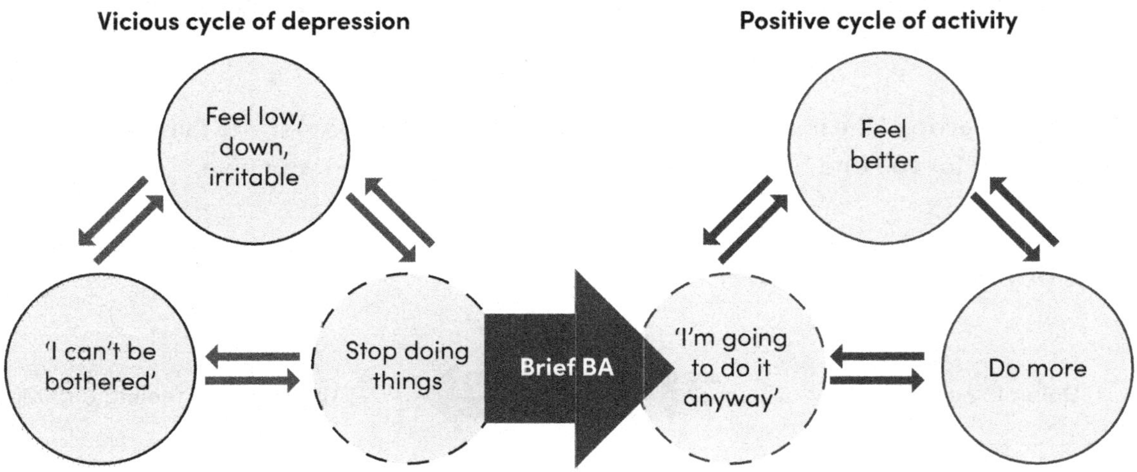

THE BRIEF BA MODEL

LAVA (Life Areas, Values and Activities)

Hobbies/fun	**Education or work**	**Family**
Physical health	**Everyday stuff**	**Friends**
Looking after myself	**The bigger picture**	**Important other(s)**

Recap: Life areas I decided to do more activities towards:

Valued activities

Recap: What key value have I been doing more towards, and how?

Value:

Activity:

Activity:

Activity:

Contracts

Recap: How has involving other people been helpful?

Problem-solving

1) Identify the problem

2) Identify solutions

3) Pros and cons of each solution

4) Select a solution

5) Plan solution

6) Do it!

7) Review

Recap: When has problem-solving been helpful?

Reviewing progress

You have achieved a lot in Brief BA, no matter how much you feel still needs to change.

You have worked hard to make changes to get where you are.

The 'Healthy Me' worksheet is a good way to recognize achievements and plan for the future.

Planning for the future

You've now learned a number of skills that can help you to feel better and get more out of life, to keep making progress and to draw on if you begin to feel down again.

- It's a good idea to keep filling in your activity log and planning, especially for the next few weeks
- Eventually, you might find that you're doing a variety of activities that fit with what is important to you in life, without having to use the forms
- You still might find it useful to review these workbooks and practise the skills if you start to feel low again
- It can help to do this with the help of someone else, like a parent
- Remember the key message:

Doing more of what matters to you helps you get more out of life.

What if I still feel depressed?

Sometimes people don't realize how much things have changed, and often there are improvements even if they aren't immediately obvious. For others it can take a bit longer for the changes you've made to start affecting your mood, and for your feelings to 'catch up'.

Keep doing valued activities in different life areas regularly, and your mood should gradually improve.

Sometimes there are things that knock you back (e.g. something bad happening in your life), but you still have the tools to make progress on your own.

We will check how you're feeling in the post-treatment review (in around one month's time), and hear from both you and your parent(s).

What if I start to feel depressed again?

You might have times in the future when you start to feel depressed, but the key is using the techniques we've covered in our work to help you feel better as soon as you notice this. No matter what has happened in the past, or what happens in the future, it's possible to make changes to your life, make the best of circumstances, and spend time doing activities that give your life purpose and meaning.

If your depression symptoms continue to significantly interfere with your life, you should speak with your family doctor.

Who can I speak to now our sessions have finished?

We will be meeting again to assess your progress since starting this treatment. Before then, contact us using the details below.

Contact:

There are also lots of ways you can get extra help once our work is over, including using the resources suggested below.

Useful resources for self-help

Books

- Dummett, N. and Williams, C. (2008) *Overcoming Teenage Low Mood and Depression: A Five Areas Approach.* London: Hodder Arnold.
- Fennell, M. (1999) *Overcoming Low Self-Esteem: A Self-Help Guide Using Cognitive Behavioural Techniques.* London: Constable & Robinson.
- Gilbert, P. (1997) *Overcoming Depression: A Self-Help Guide Using Cognitive Behavioural Techniques.* London: Constable & Robinson.
- Reynolds, S. and Parkinson, M. (2015) *Am I Depressed and What Can I Do About It? A CBT Self-Help Guide for Teenagers Experiencing Low Mood and Depression.* London: Hachette UK.
- Stallard, P. (2002) *Think Good – Feel Good: A Cognitive Behaviour Therapy Workbook for Children and Young People.* Chichester: John Wiley & Sons (plus additional online resources after purchasing the book: www.wileyeurope.com/go/thinkgoodfeelgood).

Websites

- Childline, www.childline.org.uk; if you would prefer to speak to a counsellor online, www.childline.org.uk/talk/chat/pages/onlinechat.aspx (or you can exchange emails with a counsellor)
- Harmless, a user-led organization that includes a range of information and support for people who self-harm, www.harmless.org.uk

- Living Life to the Full (LLTTF), a useful website with a range of booklets, worksheets and computer-based self-help modules, https://llttf.com
- moodgym, a free web-based CBT programme, which includes modules on assertiveness and interpersonal skills, https://moodgym.com.au
- Moodjuice, a self-help site full of resources and booklets for dealing with depression, anxiety and other difficulties, www.moodjuice.scot.nhs.uk
- PAPYRUS, Prevention of Young Suicide, advice and support for people worried about young people dealing with self-harm and emotional distress, https://papyrus-uk.org
- The Site, an online guide to life for young people aged under 25, www.themix.org.uk

Helplines

- Childline, a free confidential 24-hour helpline for young people up to the age of 19: 0800 1111
- PAPYRUS HOPELINEUK, a free confidential helpline for anyone concerned about a young person at risk of harming themselves (open weekdays 10am–5pm, 7pm–10pm; weekends 2pm–5pm): 0800 068 4141
- Samaritans, a free confidential 24-hour helpline: 116 123

Support groups

- Mind, provides information on mental health problems and treatments. Helpline 0300 123 3393 (Mon–Fri 9am–5pm), www.mind.org.uk
- Rethink, provides information and a helpline for anyone affected by mental health problems. Helpline 0300 500 0927, www.rethink.org
- Young Minds, a charity committed to improving the mental health of young people. Provides support for those worried about a young person's behaviour or mental health, and also provides information leaflets, https://youngminds.org.uk

Parent Brief BA Session 8 Worksheet

Reviewing progress

We have covered lots of topics in our Brief BA sessions, so here is a recap of the key ideas so you can think about what was most useful for your child, and how you can support them to keep these skills going after our sessions end.

Beating depression with Brief BA

1) **Doing** things differently → **LEADS TO** → 2) **Thinking** and **feeling** differently

Activity monitoring

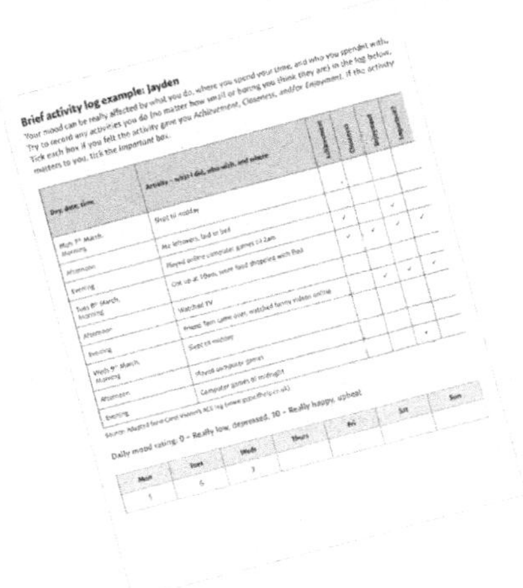

Activity monitoring

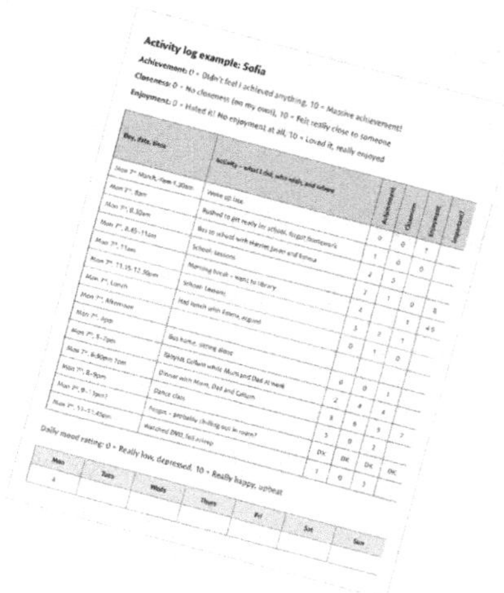

What did my child and I learn by them completing an activity log?

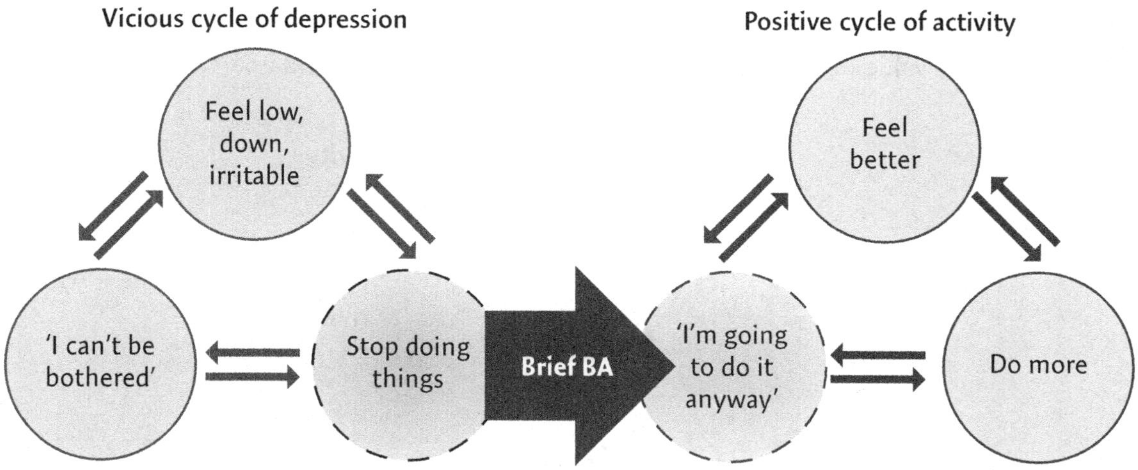

THE BRIEF BA MODEL

LAVA (Life Areas, Values and Activities)

Hobbies/fun	**Education or work**	**Family**
Physical health	**Everyday stuff**	**Friends**
Looking after myself	**The bigger picture**	**Important other(s)**

Life areas my child decided to do more activities towards:

Valued activities

Recap: What was one value my child found helpful to do more towards, and how?

Value:

Activity:

Activity:

Activity:

Contracts

How has involving other people been helpful for my child?

What has that been like for me?

Problem-solving

1) Identify the problem

2) Identify solutions

3) Pros and cons of each solution

4) Select a solution

5) Plan solution

6) Do it!

7) Review

Times when problem-solving has been helpful for my child:

Planning for the future

Your child has now learned a number of skills that can help them feel better and help them if they begin to feel down again. These points might be helpful to consider:

- It's a good idea for your child to keep filling in their activity log and LAVA worksheet, especially for the next few weeks
- Eventually, your child might find that they're doing a variety of activities that fit with what is important to them in life, without having to use the forms
- Your child still might find it useful to review these workbooks and practise the skills if they start to feel low again
- It might be useful for your child to review these worksheets with you, or someone else who can offer help
- You can also review this manual yourself and think about how you can encourage your child to continue making progress
- Remember the key message:

Doing more of what matters to you helps you get more out of life.

Your child has worked hard and achieved a lot, no matter how much they (or you) feel things still need to change. The 'Healthy Me' worksheet is a good way to recognize achievements and plan for the future. It's also useful for you to talk with your child about what they feel they have got out of Brief BA sessions, and how you can take this forwards as a family.

What if my child still feels depressed?

Sometimes people don't realize how much things have changed, and often there are improvements even if they aren't immediately obvious. Sometimes it can take a bit longer for the changes your child has made to start affecting their mood, and for their feelings to 'catch up'.

Keep encouraging your child to do valued activities across different life areas, and your child's mood should gradually improve.

Sometimes there are things that knock your child back (e.g. something bad happens in your child's life), but they still have the tools to make progress on their own. We will check how your child is feeling in the post-treatment review (in around one month's time), and hear from both your child and you.

What if my child starts to feel depressed again?

Your child might have times in the future when they start to feel depressed, but the key is using the techniques we've covered in our work to help your child feel better as soon as they notice this. No matter what has happened in the past or happens in the future, it's possible for your child to make changes to their life, make the best of circumstances, and spend time doing activities that give their life purpose and meaning.

If your child's depression symptoms continue to be significantly interfering with their life, speak to your family doctor.

Who can I speak to now our sessions have finished?

We will be meeting again in a month to assess your child's progress since starting Brief BA. Before then, contact us using the details below.

Contact:

There are also lots of ways you and your child can get extra help once our work is over, including using the resources suggested below.

Useful resources for self-help

Books

- Dummett, N. and Williams, C. (2008) *Overcoming Teenage Low Mood and Depression: A Five Areas Approach*. London: Hodder Arnold.
- Fennell, M. (1999) *Overcoming Low Self-Esteem: A Self-Help Guide Using Cognitive Behavioural Techniques*. London: Constable & Robinson.
- Gilbert, P. (1997) *Overcoming Depression: A Self-Help Guide Using Cognitive Behavioural Techniques*. London: Constable & Robinson.
- Reynolds, S. and Parkinson, M. (2015) *Am I Depressed and What Can I Do About It? A CBT Self-Help Guide for Teenagers Experiencing Low Mood and Depression*. London: Hachette UK.
- Reynolds, S. and Parkinson, M. (2015) *Teenage Depression – A CBT Guide for Parents: Help Your Child Beat Their Low Mood*. London: Hachette UK.

Websites

- Childline, www.childline.org.uk; if your child would prefer to speak to a counsellor online, www.childline.org.uk/talk/chat/pages/onlinechat.aspx (or your child can exchange emails with a counsellor)
- Harmless, a user-led organization that includes a range of information and support for people who self-harm, www.harmless.org.uk
- Living Life to the Full (LLTTF), a useful website with a range of booklets, worksheets and computer-based self-help modules, https://llttf.com

- moodgym, a free web-based CBT programme, which includes modules on assertiveness and interpersonal skills, https://moodgym.com.au
- Moodjuice, a self-help site full of resources and booklets for dealing with depression, anxiety and other difficulties, www.moodjuice.scot.nhs.uk
- PAPYRUS, Prevention of Young Suicide, advice and support for people worried about young people dealing with self-harm and emotional distress, https://papyrus-uk.org/worried-about-someone

Helplines

- Childline, a free confidential 24-hour helpline for young people up to the age of 19: 0800 1111
- PAPYRUS HOPELINEUK, a free confidential helpline for anyone concerned about a young person at risk of harming themselves (open weekdays 10am–5pm, 7pm–10pm; weekends 2pm–5pm): 0800 068 4141
- Samaritans, a free confidential 24-hour helpline: 116 123

Support groups

- Mind, provides information on mental health problems and treatments. Helpline 0300 123 3393 (Mon–Fri 9am–5pm), www.mind.org.uk
- Rethink, provides information and a helpline for anyone affected by mental health problems. Helpline 0300 5000 927, www.rethink.org

For parents and carers

- Family Lives (formerly known as Parentline), a national charity offering free support services to parents and carers. Helpline: 0808 800 2222, www.familylives.org.uk
- Young Minds, For Parents, Parents Helpline: 0808 802 5544 (free helpline, open Mon–Fri 9.30am–4pm, or chat online weekdays 11am–1pm), https://youngminds.org.uk/find-help/for-parents

Brief BA Review Checklist

ID/Client initials:

Date:

Brief BA Review Checklist *Agree with family how to split session: some time with young person and parent but also time with young person alone*	
Complete?	**Task**
	Audio/video recorder on
	Anything in particular to make time for today? Details:
	Complete ROMs: • Young person symptom questionnaire (e.g. RCADS Depression Subscale + Risk Q, or full RCADS if not done recently) • Young person functioning/quality of life questionnaire (e.g. ORS) • Parent report of young person symptom questionnaire (e.g. RCADS Depression Subscale + Risk Q, or full RCADS if not done recently) • Parent report of young person functioning/quality of life questionnaire (e.g. ORS)
	Feed back ROMs scores: graphs, what the scores mean for age/sex of client, e.g. • Full RCADS parent and young person: subscales and what they indicate in terms of clinical levels for each • ORS parent and young person • SRS parent and young person
	Review goal progress
	Review progress since Session 8
	What happens next: Agree discharge unless significant depression symptoms or risk remains
	Depending on age: • Inform family of option to re-refer to services OR: • Inform family of options to access adult services
	Inform family a summary letter will be sent to them and copy to:
	Young person service-related experience questionnaire (if applicable, e.g. Chi-ESQ)
	Parent service-related experience questionnaire (if applicable, e.g. Chi-ESQ)
	Young person session feedback questionnaire (e.g. SRS)
	Parent session feedback questionnaire (e.g. SRS)
	Goodbye

After review	
Complete?	**Task**
	Upload audio/video recording and delete from device
	Score young person and parent ROMs (if not done in session)
	Outcome electronic diary appointment (if applicable)
	Electronic or paper session record: ROMs, risk, attendees, content, treatment/discharge plan
	Upload completed session worksheets and ROMs to electronic records (if applicable)
	Diary appointment for next session
	Prepare to discuss in supervision
	Feedback to team re. outcome of Brief BA
	Send summary closing letter

References

Abramson, L.Y., Metalsky, G.I. and Alloy, L.B. (1989) 'Hopelessness depression: A theory-based subtype of depression.' *Psychological Review 96*(2), 358.

Acierno, R., Gros, D.F., Ruggiero, K.J., Hernandez-Tejada, M.A., *et al.* (2016) 'Behavioral activation and therapeutic exposure for posttraumatic stress disorder: A noninferiority trial of treatment delivered in person versus home-based telehealth.' *Depression and Anxiety 33*(5), 415–423.

Ahn, S. and Fedewa, A.L. (2011) 'A meta-analysis of the relationship between children's physical activity and mental health.' *Journal of Pediatric Psychology 36*(4), 385–397.

APA (American Psychiatric Association) (2013) *Diagnostic and Statistical Manual of Mental Disorders* (5th edn). Arlington, VA: APA.

Auerbach, R.P., Stanton, C.H., Proudfit, G.H. and Pizzagalli, D.A. (2015) 'Self-referential processing in depressed adolescents: A high-density event-related potential study.' *Journal of Abnormal Psychology 124*(2), 233.

Baddeley, A.D. and Hitch, G.J. (1994) 'Development in the concept of working memory.' *Neuropsychology 8*(4), 485.

Bandura, A. (1978) 'Social learning theory of aggression.' *Journal of Communication 28*(3), 12–29.

Beck, A.T. (1979) *Cognitive Therapy of Depression.* New York: Guilford Press.

Beck, A.T. (1983) 'Cognitive Therapy of Depression: New Perspectives.' In P.J. Clayton and J.E. Barett (eds) *Treatment of Depression: Old Controversies and New Approaches* (pp.265–284). New York: Raven Press.

Blake, M.J., Sheeber, L.B., Youssef, G.J., Raniti, M.B. and Allen, N.B. (2017) 'Systematic review and meta-analysis of adolescent cognitive-behavioral sleep interventions.' *Clinical Child and Family Psychology Review 20*(3), 227–249.

Blakemore, S.J. (2017) *Inventing Ourselves: The Secret Life of the Teenage Brain.* New York: Doubleday.

Blakemore, S.J. and Choudhury, S. (2006) 'Development of the adolescent brain: Implications for executive function and social cognition.' *Journal of Child Psychology and Psychiatry 47*(3–4), 296–312.

Blakemore, S.J. and Robbins, T.W. (2012) 'Decision-making in the adolescent brain.' *Nature Neuroscience 15*(9), 1184.

Bohn, A. and Berntsen, D. (2013) 'The future is bright and predictable: The development of prospective life stories across childhood and adolescence.' *Developmental Psychology 49*(7), 1232.

Bonete, S., Calero, M.D. and Fernández-Parra, A. (2015) 'Group training in interpersonal problem-solving skills for workplace adaptation of adolescents and adults with Asperger syndrome: A preliminary study.' *Autism 19*(4), 409–420.

Bordin, E.S. (1979) 'The generalizability of the psychoanalytic concept of the working alliance.' *Psychotherapy: Theory, Research & Practice 16*(3), 252–260.

Bozarth, J.D. (2002) 'Nondirectivity in the person-centered approach: Critique of Kahn's critique.' *Journal of Humanistic Psychology 42*(2), 78–83.

Braams, B.R., van Duijvenvoorde, A.C., Peper, J.S. and Crone, E.A. (2015) 'Longitudinal changes in adolescent risk-taking: A comprehensive study of neural responses to rewards, pubertal development, and risk-taking behavior.' *Journal of Neuroscience 35*(18), 7226–7238.

Brady, P., Kangas, M. and McGill, K. (2017) '"Family matters": A systematic review of the evidence for family psychoeducation for major depressive disorder.' *Journal of Marital and Family Therapy 43*(2), 245–263.

Brosan, L., Reynolds, S. and Moore, R.G. (2008) 'Self-evaluation of cognitive therapy performance: Do therapists know how competent they are?' *Behavioural and Cognitive Psychotherapy 36*(5), 581–587.

Burton, C., McKinstry, B., Tătar, A.S., Serrano-Blanco, A., Pagliari, C. and Wolters, M. (2013) 'Activity monitoring in patients with depression: A systematic review.' *Journal of Affective Disorders 145*(1), 21–28.

Chorpita, B.F., Yim, L., Moffitt, C., Umemoto, L.A. and Francis, S.E. (2000) 'Assessment of symptoms of DSM-IV anxiety and depression in children: A revised child anxiety and depression scale.' *Behaviour Research and Therapy 38*, 835–855. doi:10.1016/S0005-7967(99)00130-8.

Choudhury, S., Blakemore, S.J. and Charman, T. (2006) 'Social cognitive development during adolescence.' *Social Cognitive and Affective Neuroscience 1*(3), 165–174.

Chu, B.C., Crocco, S.T., Esseling, P., Areizaga, M.J., *et al.* (2016) 'Transdiagnostic group behavioral activation and exposure therapy for youth anxiety and depression: Initial randomized controlled trial.' *Behaviour Research and Therapy 76*, 65–75.

Clark, D.A. and Oates, T. (1995) 'Daily hassles, major and minor life events, and their interaction with sociotropy and autonomy.' *Behaviour Research and Therapy 33*(7), 819–823.

Connolly, S.L., Abramson, L.Y. and Alloy, L.B. (2016) 'Information processing biases concurrently and prospectively predict depressive symptoms in adolescents: Evidence from a self-referent encoding task.' *Cognition and Emotion 30*(3), 550–560. doi:10.1080/02699931.2015.1010488.

Conway, M. (2005) 'Memory and the self.' *Journal of Memory and Language 53*(4), 594–628. doi:10.1016/j.jml.2005.08.005.

Conway, M. and Pleydell-Pearce, C.W. (2000) 'The construction of autobiographical memories in the self-memory system.' *Psychological Review 107*(2), 261–288. doi:10.1037//0033-295x.

Costello, J.E., and Angold, A. (1988) 'Scales to assess child and adolescent depression – Checklists, screens and nets.' *Journal of the American Academy of Child and Adolescent Psychiatry 27*, 726–737.

Cottrell, D. and Boston, P. (2002) 'Practitioner review: The effectiveness of systemic family therapy for children and adolescents.' *Journal of Child Psychology and Psychiatry 43*(5), 573–586.

Cox, L.J., Stanley, B.H., Melhem, N.M., Oquendo, M.A., *et al.* (2012) 'A longitudinal study of nonsuicidal self-injury in offspring at high risk for mood disorder.' *The Journal of Clinical Psychiatry 73*(6), 821.

Cuijpers, P., van Straten, A. and Warmerdam, E.H. (2007) 'Behavioral treatment of depression: A meta-analysis of activity scheduling.' *Clinical Psychology Review 27*(3), 318–326.

Damon, W. and Hart, D. (1988) *Self-Understanding in Childhood and Adolescence.* New York: Cambridge University Press.

DeCou, C.R. and Schumann, M.E. (2018) 'On the iatrogenic risk of assessing suicidality: A meta-analysis.' *Suicide and Life-Threatening Behavior 48*(5), 531–543.

Donahue, E.M., Robins, R.W., Roberts, B.W. and John, O.P. (1993) 'The divided self: Concurrent and longitudinal effects of psychological adjustment and social roles on self-concept differentiation.' *Journal of Personality and Social Psychology 64*(5), 834–846.

Duncan, B.L., Miller, S.D., Sparks, J.A., Claud, D.A., *et al.* (2003) 'The Session Rating Scale: Preliminary psychometric properties of a "working" alliance measure.' *Journal of Brief Therapy 3*(1), 3–12.

D'Zurilla, T.J. and Nezu, A.M. (1986) *Problem-Solving Therapy: A Social Competence Approach to Clinical Intervention* (Vol. 18). New York: Springer.

Edbrooke-Childs, J., Wolpert, M. and Deighton, J. (2016) 'Using patient reported outcome measures to improve service effectiveness (UPROMISE): Training clinicians to use outcome measures in child mental health.' *Administration and Policy in Mental Health and Mental Health Services Research 43*(3), 302–308.

Ekers, D., Godfrey, C., Gilbody, S., Parrott, S., *et al.* (2011) 'Cost utility of behavioural activation delivered by the non-specialist.' *The British Journal of Psychiatry 199*, 510–511.

Ekers, D., Webster, L., Van Straten, A., Cuijpers, P., Richards, D. and Gilbody, S. (2014) 'Behavioural activation for depression: An update of meta-analysis of effectiveness and sub group analysis.' *PLoS ONE 9*(6), e100100. doi:10.1371/journal.pone.0100100.

Emmelkamp, P., van der Helm, M., MacGillavry, D. and van Zanten, B. (1984) 'Marital Therapy with Clinically Distressed Couples: A Comparative Evaluation of System-Theoretic, Contingency Contracting, and Communication Skills Approaches.' In K. Hahlweg and N.S. Jacobson (eds) *Marital Interaction: Analysis and Modification* (pp.36–52). New York: Guilford Press.

Falloon, I.R. (1991) 'Behavioral family therapy.' *Handbook of Family Therapy 2*, 65–95.

Ferrey, A.E., Hughes, N.D., Simkin, S., Locock, L., *et al.* (2016) 'The impact of self-harm by young people on parents and families: A qualitative study.' *BMJ Open 6*(1), e009631.

Fisk, J., Ellis, J.A. and Reynolds, S.A. (2019) 'A test of the CaR-FA-X mechanisms and depression in adolescents.' *Memory 27*(4), 455–464.

Fluckiger, C., Del Re, A.C., Wampold, B. and Horvath, A.O. (2018) 'The alliance in adult psychotherapy: A meta-analysis synthesis.' *Psychotherapy 55*, 316–340.

Forbes, E.E., Ryan, N.D., Phillips, M.L., Manuck, S.B., *et al.* (2010) 'Healthy adolescents' neural response to reward: associations with puberty, positive affect, and depressive symptoms.' *Journal of the American Academy of Child & Adolescent Psychiatry 49*(2), 162–172.

Fox, K.R., Franklin, J.C., Ribeiro, J.D., Kleiman, E.M., Bentley, K.H. and Nock, M.K. (2015) 'Meta-analysis of risk factors for nonsuicidal self-injury.' *Clinical Psychology Review 42*, 156–167.

Gathercole, S.E. and Alloway, T.P. (2008) *Working Memory and Learning: A Practical Guide for Teachers.* London: Sage.

Gillon, E. (2007) 'An introduction to person-centred counselling psychology.' Available at: www.firstpsychology.co.uk/files/person_centred_theory.pdf

Goldfried, M.R. (2007) 'What has psychotherapy inherited from Carl Rogers?' *Psychotherapy: Theory, Research, Practice, Training 44*, 3, 249–325. doi:10.1037/0033-3204.44.3.249.

Gondek, D., Edbrooke-Childs, J., Fink, E., Deighton, J. and Wolpert, M. (2016) 'Feedback from outcome measures and treatment effectiveness, treatment efficiency, and collaborative practice: A systematic review.' *Administration and Policy in Mental Health 43*, 325–343. Available at: https://doi.org/10.1007/s10488-015-0710-5

Goodyer, I.M., Herbert, J., Tamplin, A. and Altham, P.M.E. (2000) 'Recent life events, cortisol, dehydroepiandrosterone and the onset of major depression in high-risk adolescents.' *The British Journal of Psychiatry 177*(6), 499–504.

Goodyer, I.M., Reynolds, S., Barrett, B., Byford, S., *et al.* (2017) 'Cognitive behavioural therapy and short-term psychoanalytical psychotherapy versus a brief psychosocial intervention in adolescents with unipolar major depressive disorder (IMPACT): A multicentre, pragmatic, observer-blind, randomised controlled superiority trial.' *The Lancet Psychiatry 4*(2), 109–119.

Guffanti, G., Gameroff, M.J., Warner, V., Talati, A., *et al.* (2016) 'Heritability of major depressive and comorbid anxiety disorders in multi-generational families at high risk for depression.' *American Journal of Medical Genetics Part B: Neuropsychiatric Genetics 171*(8), 1072–1079.

Gustavson, K.A., Alexopoulos, G.S., Niu, G.C., McCulloch, C., Meade, T. and Areán, P.A. (2016) 'Problem-solving therapy reduces suicidal ideation in depressed older adults with executive dysfunction.' *The American Journal of Geriatric Psychiatry 24*(1), 11–17.

Hards, E., Ellis, J., Fisk, J. and Reynolds, S. (2019a) 'Memories of the self in adolescence: Examining 6558 self-image norms.' *Memory*, 1–7.

Hards, E., Ellis, J., Fisk, J. and Reynolds, S. (2019b) 'Negative view of the self and symptoms of depression in adolescents.' *Journal of Affective Disorders, 262*(1), 143–148.

Hart, R.R. (1978) 'Therapeutic effectiveness of setting and monitoring goals.' *Journal of Consulting and Clinical Psychology 46*(6), 1242.

Harter, S. (1998) 'The Development of Self-Representations.' In W. Damon and N. Eisenberg (eds) *Handbook of Child Psychology: Vol. 3. Social, Emotional and Personality Development* (5th edn) (pp.553–617). New York: Wiley.

Harter, S. (2006) 'The Self.' In N. Eisenberg, E. Damon and R.M. Lerner (eds) *Handbook of Child Psychology: Social, Emotional, and Personality Development* (6th edn) (pp.505–561). Hoboken, NJ: John Wiley & Sons.

Harter, S. (2012) *The Construction of the Self* (2nd edn). New York: Guilford Press.

Heath, N.L., Carsley, D., De Riggi, M.E., Mills, D. and Mettler, J. (2016) 'The relationship between mindfulness, depressive symptoms, and non-suicidal self-injury amongst adolescents.' *Archives of Suicide Research 20*(4), 635–649.

Hooker, S.A., Slattengren, A.H., Boyle, L. and Sherman, M.D. (2019) 'Values-based behavioral activation for chronic pain in primary care: A pilot study.' *Journal of Clinical Psychology in Medical Settings*, 1–10.

Horvath, A.O. and Luborsky, L. (1993) 'The role of the therapeutic alliance in psychotherapy.' *Journal of Consulting and Clinical Psychology 61*, 561–573.

Horwitz, A.G., Berona, J., Czyz, E.K., Yeguez, C.E. and King, C.A. (2017) 'Positive and negative expectations of hopelessness as longitudinal predictors of depression, suicidal ideation, and suicidal behavior in high-risk adolescents.' *Suicide and Life-Threatening Behavior 47*(2), 168–176.

IMPACT (Improving Mood with Psychoanalytic and Cognitive Therapies) (2010) *Cognitive Behaviour Therapy for Depression in Young People: Manual for Therapists*. Cambridge: IMPACT Trial Office. Available at: http://dev.psychiatry.cam.ac.uk/files/2016/06/CBT-Manual.pdf

Jacka, F.N., O'Neil, A., Opie, R., Itsiopoulos, C., *et al.* (2017) 'A randomised controlled trial of dietary improvement for adults with major depression (the "SMILES" trial).' *BMC Medicine 15*, 23. Available at: http://doi.org/10.1186/s12916-017-0791-y

Jacobson, N.S., Dobson, K.S., Truax, P.A., Addis, M.E., *et al.* (1996) 'A component analysis of cognitive-behavioral treatment for depression.' *Journal of Consulting and Clinical Psychology 64*(2), 295–304.

Jahoda, A., Hastings, R., Hatton, C., Cooper, S.A., *et al.* (2017) 'Comparison of behavioural activation with guided self-help for treatment of depression in adults with intellectual disabilities: A randomised controlled trial.' *The Lancet Psychiatry 4*(12), 909–919.

Jones, R.B., Thapar, A., Stone, Z., Thapar, A., *et al.* (2018) 'Psychoeducational interventions in adolescent depression: A systematic review.' *Patient Education and Counseling 101*(5), 804–816.

Karver, M.S., De Nadai, A.S., Monahan, M. and Shirk, S.R. (2018) 'Meta-analysis of the prospective relation between alliance and outcome in child and adolescent psychotherapy.' *Psychotherapy 55*(4), 341–355.

Kauer, S.D., Reid, S.C., Crooke, A.H.D., Khor, A., *et al.* (2012) 'Self-monitoring using mobile phones in the early stages of adolescent depression: randomized controlled trial.' *Journal of Medical Internet Research 14*(3), e67.

Kaufman, J., Birmaher, B., Brent, D., Rao, U., *et al.* (1997) 'Schedule for affective disorders and schizophrenia for school-age children-present and lifetime version (K-SADS-PL): Initial reliability and validity data.' *Journal of the American Academy of Child & Adolescent Psychiatry 36*(7), 980–988. Available at: https://doi.org/10.1097/00004583-199707000-00021

Kendrick, T., El-Gohary, M., Stuart, B., Gilbody, S., *et al.* (2016) 'Routine use of patient reported outcome measures (PROMS) for improving treatment of common mental health problems in adults.' *Cochrane Database of Systematic Reviews 7*. doi:1002/14651858.CD011119.pub2.

Khalid, S., Williams, C. and Reynolds, S. (2016) 'Is there an association between diet and depression in children and adolescents? A systematic review.' *British Journal of Nutrition 116*, 2097–2108. doi:10 1017/S0007114516004359.

Knox, M., Funk, J., Elliot, R. and Bush, E.G. (1998) 'Adolescents' possible selves and their relationship to global self-esteem.' *Sex Roles 39*(1–2), 61–80.

Kokkevi, A., Rotsika, V., Arapaki, A. and Richardson, C. (2012) 'Adolescents' self-reported suicide attempts, self-harm thoughts and their correlates across 17 European countries.' *Journal of Child Psychology and Psychiatry 53*(4), 381–389.

Kouros, C.D. and Garber, J. (2014) 'Trajectories of individual depressive symptoms in adolescents: Gender and family relationships as predictors.' *Developmental Psychology 50*(12), 2633.

Law, D. and Jacob, J. (2015) *Goals and Goal Based Outcomes (GBOs): Some Useful Information* (3rd edn). London: CAMHS Press.

Lejuez, C.W., Hopko, D.R. and Hopko, S.D. (2001) 'A brief behavioral activation treatment for depression: Treatment manual.' *Behavior Modification 25*, 255–286.

Lejuez, C.W., Hopko, D.R., Acierno, R., Daughters, S.B. and Pagoto, S.L. (2011) 'Ten year revision of the brief behavioral activation treatment for depression: Revised treatment manual.' *Behavior Modification 35*, 111–161.

Lewinsohn, P.M. (1974) 'A Behavioral Approach to Depression.' In R.J. Friedman and M.M. Katz (eds) *Psychology of Depression: Contemporary Theory and Research* (pp.157–178). Oxford: Wiley.

Maddox, L. (2018) *Blueprint: How Our Childhood Makes Us Who We Are*. London: Robinson.

Markus, H. and Nurius, P. (1986) 'Possible selves.' *American Psychologist 41*(9), 954–969. doi:10.1037/0003-066X.41.9.954.

Martell, C.R., Addis, M.E. and Jacobson, N.S. (2001) *Depression in Context: Strategies for Guided Action*. New York: W. W. Norton & Co.

Martin, F. and Oliver, T. (2018) 'Behavioural activation for children and young people: A systematic review of progress and promise.' *European Child & Adolescent Psychiatry 28*, 427–441. Available at: https://doi.org/10.1007/s00787-018-1126-z

Mathias, C.W., Michael Furr, R., Sheftall, A.H., Hill-Kapturczak, N., Crum, P. and Dougherty, D.M. (2012) 'What's the harm in asking about suicidal ideation?' *Suicide and Life-Threatening Behavior 42*(3), 341–351.

McCall, W.V., Blocker, J.N., D'Agostino Jr, R., Kimball, J., *et al.* (2010) 'Insomnia severity is an indicator of suicidal ideation during a depression clinical trial.' *Sleep Medicine 11*(9), 822–827.

McCauley, E., Gudmundsen, G., Schloredt, K., Martell, C., *et al.* (2016) 'The adolescent behavioral activation program: Adapting behavioral activation as a treatment for depression in adolescence.' *Journal of Clinical Child & Adolescent Psychology 45*(3), 291–304.

McCay, E., Beanlands, H., Leszcz, M., Goering, P., *et al.* (2006) 'A group intervention to promote healthy self-concepts and guide recovery in first episode schizophrenia: A pilot study.' *Psychiatric Rehabilitation Journal 30*(2), 105.

McHugh, C.M., Lee, R.S.C., Hermens, D.F., Corderoy, A., Large, M. and Hickie, I.B. (2019) 'Impulsivity in the self-harm and suicidal behavior of young people: A systematic review and meta-analysis.' *Journal of Psychiatric Research 116*, 51–60.

McMakin, D.L., Olino, T.M., Porta, G., Dietz, L.J., *et al.* (2012) 'Anhedonia predicts poorer recovery among youth with selective serotonin reuptake inhibitor treatment-resistant depression.' *Journal of the American Academy of Child & Adolescent Psychiatry 51*(4), 404–411.

Miller, S.D. and Duncan, B.L. (2000) 'Outcome rating scale (ORS).' Available at: https://scott-d-miller-ph-d.myshopify.com/collections/performance-metrics/products/performance-metrics-licenses-for-the-ors-and-srs

Morgan, C., Webb, R.T., Carr, M.J., Kontopantelis, E., *et al.* (2017) 'Incidence, clinical management, and mortality risk following self harm among children and adolescents: Cohort study in primary care.' *BMJ 359*, j4351.

Mufson, L., Moreau, D., Weissman, M.M. and Klerman, G.L. (2015) *Interpersonal Psychotherapy for Depressed Adolescents*. New York: Guilford Press.

Murakami, K. and Sasaki, S. (2010) 'Dietary intake and depressive symptoms: A systematic review of observational studies.' *Molecular Nutrition & Food Research 54*(4), 471–488. Available at: http://doi.org/10.1002/mnfr.200900157

Nezu, A.M., Nezu, C.M. and Perri, M.G. (1989) *Problem Solving Therapy for Depression: Theory Research and Clinical Guidelines*. Oxford: John Wiley & Sons.

NICE (National Institute for Health and Care Excellence) (2019) *Depression in Children and Young People: Identification and Management*. NG134. Available at: www.nice.org.uk/guidance/ng134/resources/depression-in-children-and-young-people-identification-and-management-pdf-66141719350981

O'Keeffe, S., Martin, P., Target, M. and Midgley, N. (2019) '"I just stopped going": A mixed methods investigation into types of therapy dropout in adolescents with depression.' *Frontiers in Psychology 10*, 75.

O'Mahen, H.A., Woodford, J., McGinley, J., Warren, F.C., *et al.* (2013) 'Internet-based behavioral activation – Treatment for postnatal depression (Netmums): A randomized controlled trial.' *Journal of Affective Disorders 150*(3), 814–822.

O'Neill, J. (2000) 'SMART goals, SMART schools.' *Educational Leadership 57*(5), 46–50.

ONS (Office for National Statistics) (2016) 'Top 5 leading causes of death by sex and five-year age group, England and Wales: 2014 registrations.' Available at: www.ons.gov.uk/peoplepopulationandcommunity/birthsdeathsandmarriages/deaths/adhocs/005656top5leading causesofdeathbysexandfiveyearagegroupengland andwales 2014registrations

ONS (2019) 'Suicides in the UK: 2018 registrations.' Available at: www.ons.gov.uk/releases/suicidesintheuk2018registrations

Orchard, F., Pass, L., Marshall, T. and Reynolds, S. (2017) 'Clinical characteristics of adolescents referred for treatment of depressive disorders.' *Child and Adolescent Mental Health 22*(2), 61–68.

Orchard, F., Pass, L. and Reynolds, S. (2019) '"I am worthless and kind": The specificity of positive and negative self-evaluation in adolescent depression.' *British Journal of Clinical Psychology 58*(3), 260–273.

Orchard, F. and Reynolds, S. (2018) 'The combined influence of cognitions in adolescent depression: Biases of interpretation, self-evaluation, and memory.' *British Journal of Clinical Psychology 57*(4), 420–435.

Owens, C., Hansford, L., Sharkey, S. and Ford, T. (2016) 'Needs and fears of young people presenting at accident and emergency department following an act of self-harm: Secondary analysis of qualitative data.' *The British Journal of Psychiatry 208*(3), 286–291.

Oyserman, D., Bybee, D., Terry, K. and Hart-Johnson, T. (2004) 'Possible selves as roadmaps.' *Journal of Research in Personality 38*(2), 130–149.

Packard, B.W.L. and Conway, P.F. (2006) 'Methodological choice and its consequences for possible selves research.' *Identity 6*(3), 251–271.

Pass, L., Hodgson, E., Whitney, H. and Reynolds, S. (2018) 'Brief behavioral activation treatment for depressed adolescents delivered by nonspecialist clinicians: A case illustration.' *Cognitive and Behavioral Practice 25*(2), 208–224.

Pass, L., Lejuez, C.W. and Reynolds, S. (2018) 'Brief behavioural activation (Brief BA) for adolescent depression: A pilot study.' *Behavioural and Cognitive Psychotherapy 46*(2), 182–194.

Pass, L., Sancho, M., Brett, S., Jones, M. and Reynolds, S. (2018) 'Brief Behavioural Activation (Brief BA) in secondary schools: A feasibility study examining acceptability and practical considerations.' *Educational and Child Psychology 35*(2).

Pass, L., Whitney, H. and Reynolds, S. (2016) 'Brief behavioral activation for adolescent depression: Working with complexity and risk.' *Clinical Case Studies 15*(5), 360–375.

Pasterfield, M., Bailey, D., Hems, D., McMillan, D., Richards, D. and Gilbody, S. (2014) 'Adapting manualized behavioural activation treatment for older adults with depression.' *The Cognitive Behaviour Therapist 7*.

Pizzagalli, D.A. (2014) 'Depression, stress, and anhedonia: Toward a synthesis and integrated model.' *Annual Review of Clinical Psychology 10*, 393–423.

Polanczyk, G.V., Salum, G.A., Sugaya, L.S., Caye, A. and Rohde, L.A. (2015) 'Annual Research Review: A meta-analysis of the worldwide prevalence of mental disorders in children and adolescents.' *Journal of Child Psychology and Psychiatry 56*(3), 345–365.

Porter, J.F., Spates, C.R. and Smitham, S. (2004) 'Behavioral activation group therapy in public mental health settings: A pilot investigation.' *Professional Psychology: Research and Practice 35*, 297–301.

Puspitasari, A., Kanter, J. W., Murphy, J., Crowe, A. and Koerner, K. (2013) 'Developing an online, modular, active learning training program for Behavioral Activation.' *Psychotherapy: Research, Theory, Practice, Training 50*, 256–265.

Ramnerö, J., Folke, F. and Kanter, J.W. (2016) 'A learning theory account of depression.' *Scandinavian Journal of Psychology 57*(1), 73–82.

Rehm, L.P. and Plakosh, P. (1975) 'Preference for immediate reinforcement in depression.' *Journal of Behavior Therapy and Experimental Psychiatry 6*(2), 101–103.

Richards, D.A., Ekers, D., McMillan, D., Taylor, R.S., *et al.* (2016) 'Cost and Outcome of Behavioural Activation versus Cognitive Behavioural Therapy for Depression (COBRA): A randomised, controlled, non-inferiority trial.' *The Lancet 388*(10047), 871–880.

Rodway, C., Tham, S.G., Ibrahim, S., Turnbull, P., *et al.* (2016) 'Suicide in children and young people in England: A consecutive case series.' *The Lancet Psychiatry 3*(8), 751–759.

Rogers, C.R. (1951) *Client-Centered Therapy*. Boston, MA: Houghton Mifflin.

Rogers, C.R. (1965) 'The therapeutic relationship: Recent theory and research.' *Australian Journal of Psychology 17*(2), 95–108. doi:10.1080/00049536508255531.

Rømer Thomsen, K. (2015) 'Measuring anhedonia: Impaired ability to pursue, experience, and learn about reward.' *Frontiers in Psychology 6*, 1409.

Rubin, D.C. and Schulkind, M.D. (1997) 'The distribution of autobiographical memories across the lifespan.' *Memory & Cognition 25*(6), 859–866. doi:10.3758/BF03211330.

Rubin, D.C., Wetzler, S.E. and Nebes, R.D. (1986) 'Autobiographical Memory Across the Adult Lifespan.' In D.C. Rubin (ed.) *Autobiographical Memory* (pp.202–221). New York: Cambridge University Press.

Ryba, M.M., Lejuez, C.W. and Hopko, D.R. (2014) 'Behavioral activation for depressed breast cancer patients: The impact of therapeutic compliance and quantity of activities completed on symptom reduction.' *Journal of Consulting and Clinical Psychology 82*, 325–335.

Rzepa, E., Fisk, J. and McCabe, C. (2017) 'Blunted neural response to anticipation, effort and consummation of reward and aversion in adolescents with depression symptomatology.' *Journal of Psychopharmacology 31*(3), 303–311.

Sanders, M.R., Dadds, M.R., Johnston, B.M. and Cash, R. (1992) 'Childhood depression and conduct disorder: I. Behavioral, affective, and cognitive aspects of family problem-solving interactions.' *Journal of Abnormal Psychology 101*(3), 495.

Sanford, M., Boyle, M., McCleary, L., Miller, J., *et al.* (2006) 'A pilot study of adjunctive family psychoeducation in adolescent major depression: Feasibility and treatment effect.' *Journal of the American Academy of Child and Adolescent Psychiatry 45*(4), 386–395. doi:10.1097/01.chi.0000198595.68820.10.

Saunders, K.E., Hawton, K., Fortune, S. and Farrell, S. (2012) 'Attitudes and knowledge of clinical staff regarding people who self-harm: A systematic review.' *Journal of Affective Disorders 139*(3), 205–216.

Schuch, F.B., Vancampfort, D., Firth, J., Rosenbaum, S., *et al.* (2018) 'Physical activity and incident depression: A meta-analysis of prospective cohort studies.' *American Journal of Psychiatry 175*(7), 631–648.

Sedgwick, R. and Ougrin, D. (2019) 'No better than chance? Developments in predicting adolescent suicide, a commentary on Mars *et al.* (2018) and Beckman *et al.* (2018).' *Journal of Child Psychology and Psychiatry 60*(1), 100–101.

Sheeber, L., Hops, H. and Davis, B. (2001) 'Family processes in adolescent depression.' *Clinical Child and Family Psychology Review 4*(1), 19–35.

Skinner, B.F. (1938) *The Behaviour of Organisms: An Experimental Analysis.* New York: Appleton.

Singareddy, R., Krishnamurthy, V.B., Vgontzas, A.N., Fernandez-Mendoza, J., *et al.* (2013) 'Subjective and objective sleep and self-harm behaviors in young children: A general population study.' *Psychiatry Research 209*(3), 549–553.

Singer, J.A. and Salovey, A.P. (1993) *The Remembered Self.* New York: The Free Press.

Somerville, L.H. (2013) 'The teenage brain: Sensitivity to social evaluation.' *Current Directions in Psychological Science 22*(2), 121–127.

Somerville, L.H., Jones, R.M., Ruberry, E.J., Dyke, J.P., Glover, G. and Casey, B.J. (2013) 'The medial prefrontal cortex and the emergence of self-conscious emotion in adolescence.' *Psychological Science 24*(8), 1554–1562.

Spielman, A. and Anderson, M. (1999) 'The clinical interview and treatment planning as a guide to understanding the nature of insomnia: The CCNY Insomnia Interview.' *Sleep Disorders Medicine: Basic Science, Technical Considerations, and Clinical Aspects*, 385–416.

Stark, K.D., Humphrey, L.L., Crook, K. and Lewis, K. (1990) 'Perceived family environments of depressed and anxious children: Child's and maternal figure's perspectives.' *Journal of Abnormal Child Psychology 18*(5), 527–547.

St Clair-Thompson, H.L. and Gathercole, S.E. (2006) 'Executive functions and achievements in school: Shifting, updating, inhibition, and working memory.' *Quarterly Journal of Experimental Psychology 59*(4), 745–759.

Stuart, R.B. (1971) 'Behavioral contracting within the families of delinquents.' *Journal of Behavior Therapy and Experimental Psychiatry 2*(1), 1–11.

Strauss, K., Griffin, M.A. and Parker, S.K. (2012) 'Future work selves: How salient hoped-for identities motivate proactive career behaviors.' *Journal of Applied Psychology 97*(3), 580.

Tan, E., Healey, D., Gray, A.R. and Galland, B.C. (2012) 'Sleep hygiene intervention for youth aged 10 to 18 years with problematic sleep: A before-after pilot study.' *BMC Pediatrics 12*(1), 189.

Taylor, S.E., Pham, L.B., Rivkin, I.D. and Armor, D.A. (1998) 'Harnessing the imagination: Mental simulation, self-regulation, and coping.' *American Psychologist 53*(4), 429.

Timbremont, B. and Braet, C. (2006) 'Brief report: A longitudinal investigation of the relation between a negative cognitive triad and depressive symptoms in youth.' *Journal of Adolescence 29*(3), 453–458.

Tindall, L., Mikocka-Walus, A., McMillan, D., Wright, B., Hewitt, C. and Gascoyne, S. (2017) 'Is behavioural activation effective in the treatment of depression in young people? A systematic review and meta-analysis.' *Psychology and Psychotherapy: Theory, Research and Practice 90*(4), 770–796.

Tryon, G.S. and Winograd, G. (2002) 'Goal Consensus and Collaboration.' In J.C. Norcross (ed.) *Psychotherapy Relationships that Work: Therapist Contributions and Responsiveness of Patients* (pp.3–16). New York: Oxford University Press.

Vecchione, M., Alessandri, G., Roccas, S. and Caprara, G.V. (2019) 'A look into the relationship between personality traits and basic values: A longitudinal investigation.' *Journal of Personality 87*(2), 413–427.

Wade, S.L., Taylor, H.G., Yeates, K.O., Kirkwood, M., *et al.* (2018) 'Online problem solving for adolescent brain injury: A randomized trial of 2 approaches.' *Journal of Developmental & Behavioral Pediatrics 39*(2), 154–162.

Walfish, S., McAllister B., O'Donnell, P. and Lambert, M.J. (2012) 'An investigation of self-assessment bias in mental health providers.' *Psychological Reports 110*, 639–644.

Warren, J.S., Nelson, P.L., Mondragon, S.A., Baldwin, S.A. and Burlingame, G.M. (2010) 'Youth psychotherapy change trajectories and outcomes in usual care: Community mental health versus managed care settings.' *Journal of Consulting and Clinical Psychology 78*, 144–155.

Watson, R., Harvey, K., McCabe, C. and Reynolds, S. (2019) 'Understanding anhedonia: A qualitative study exploring loss of interest and pleasure in adolescent depression.' *European Child & Adolescent Psychiatry*, 1–11.

Weisz, J.R., Chorpita, B.F., Frye, A., Ng, M.Y., *et al.* (2011) 'Youth top problems: Using idiographic, consumer-guided assessment to identify treatment needs and to track change during psychotherapy.' *Journal of Consulting and Clinical Psychology 79*(3), 369–380.

Weisz, J.R., Kuppens, S., Ng, M.Y., Eckshtain, D., *et al.* (2017) 'What five decades of research tells us about the effects of youth psychological therapy: A multilevel meta-analysis and implications for science and practice.' *American Psychologist 72*(2), 79.

WHO (World Health Organization) (1992) *10: International Statistical Classification of Diseases and Related Health Problems (ICD).* Geneva: WHO.

Wilson, A.E., Buehler, R., Lawford, H., Schmidt, C. and Yong, A.G. (2012) 'Basking in projected glory: The role of subjective temporal distance in future self-appraisal.' *European Journal of Social Psychology 42*(3), 342–353.

Wollburg, E. and Braukhaus, C. (2010) 'Goal setting in psychotherapy: The relevance of approach and avoidance goals for treatment outcome.' *Psychotherapy Research 20*(4), 488–494.

Further Reading and Resources

NICE (National Institute for Health and Care Excellence) (2019) *Depression in Children and Young People: Identification and Management*. Available at: www.nice.org.uk/guidance/ng134

Reynolds, S. and Parkinson, M. (2015) *Am I Depressed and What Can I Do About It? A CBT Self-Help Guide for Teenagers Experiencing Low Mood and Depression*. London: Hachette UK.

Reynolds, S. and Parkinson, M. (2015) *Teenage Depression – A CBT Guide for Parents: Help Your Child Beat Their Low Mood*. London: Hachette UK.

Get Self Help, useful website for lots of therapist resources: www.getselfhelp.co.uk

Subject Index

Author Index

Made in the USA
Las Vegas, NV
17 November 2021

34658256R00151